Love To Lose

Love To Lose

Love Your Life and
Watch the Weight Lose Itself

Camille Martin, RD

Book cover design by Malina Jacobowitz

Published and printed in the United States by
Kindle Direct Publishing, Seattle, Washington

ISBN 978-0-578-64054-9
1. Dieting.   2. Nutrition.   3. Self-help.   4. Motivation and goal setting.
5.Women's health.   I. Title

Love To Lose
Love Your Life | Lose the Weight
camillemartinrd.com

For Sophie and Penny
Everything I do is for you.

Table of Contents

Introduction

Losing weight isn't hard — we make it hard.

I can safely say this from my own experiences in trying to lose weight. In fact, I tried to lose the same ten pounds for nearly 25 years, and the failures I endured drained my confidence to the point that I no longer saw my failures as something that happened to me — the failures *were* me.

Nothing could have been further from the truth, and if you can relate to this, the same is true for you. You most definitely are not a failure — it's your approach that is.

For some reason, our society is obsessed with the magic bullet, the one thing that will finally lead us to the Holy Grail: weight loss. But the big lie is that we believe that if we could just lose weight, our lives would be perfect. If you believe this — like I did for so many years — you've got it all wrong.

Focusing on the number on your scale, obsessing about the way your body looks, and endlessly manipulating the foods you eat keeps you from solving the real problem. The weight is only a symptom — the problem is the way you eat.

But the biggest problem, as you'll see as this book unfolds, is that by spending your life dieting, not only will you not lose weight, you'll waste your entire life stuck in a limited existence where you dumb yourself down, silence your authentic voice, and never become who you were truly meant to be.

But before we get ahead of ourselves, know this: as long as you keep dieting, nothing will change — you will never lose weight. Dieting keeps you stuck, attacking the symptom (the weight) but never solving the problem (how you eat). Not only that, dieting actually makes the problem worse. It creates massive resistance, and this resistance pushes you to keep eating in a disordered way. So you stay stuck in a vicious cycle, never making progress and blaming yourself for all the failures.

Dieting keeps you buying the winning lottery ticket, only to lose week after week. And it makes you believe that it's your fault you didn't get the right numbers.

Does chasing one diet after the next and failing over and over again sound like you? It sounds like me — or at least it did. It wasn't until I finally figured out that the weight wasn't the issue that I was finally able to lose it.

The most devastating thing about all my diet failures was that I blamed myself. If I just had more willpower, if I could just stop eating, if I could just work harder — I would finally be able to stick to a diet and lose the weight.

But that was never going to happen, because until I started getting to the source of the problem and stop attacking the symptom of it, I was going to continue to fail. And I was going to keep buying into the idea of the magic pill that would finally work, never realizing that there's no such thing.

This was me for a very long time, and if you're reading this book, I'm guessing it's you, too. But it doesn't have to be.

Once you really get to the source of the problem and address that, then you can get out of the cycle and not only stop living the miserable existence it creates but also see how much power you really have (and have had all this time) and what you're truly capable of.

I know you've heard that diets don't work, but that's only part of the equation. This book will show you exactly why they don't work, but it will also show you what does. It will also show you how forgetting about losing weight entirely — ironically — will help you lose it and how creating a bigger and better goal for yourself will speed up the process. Finally, and most importantly, it will show you that your life is so much bigger than what you look like or how much you weigh.

The biggest reason we stay stuck for so long is that we completely forget who we really are. We have an unlimited amount of inner power that has gone untapped for so long that we don't even remember that it's there. And because this power remains hidden — getting buried deeper and deeper the longer it's ignored — our voices shrink to match. Then we begin living such small lives that we don't even realize that we're not really living at all.

All of this shoving down is a huge problem. Because when you live like this for too long (like I did), it starts to feel normal. And when everyone around you is doing the same thing, it starts to look normal, too.

If you've been waiting to live your life until you lose weight — if you're skipping your high school reunion this year because you don't look as good as you want to, if you're waiting to book that trip to Hawaii until you can wear a bikini, if you refuse to get in the family photo until you look perfect — you have it all backwards. Because waiting to do these things until you lose weight is keeping you from ever losing it.

5

But once you reverse the equation, when you start really living first, the weight will come off. You don't lose weight and then do all the things you dream of doing — you fully engage in life and then watch the weight lose itself.

I've learned all of these things from experience — a painful, confidence-draining experience. And I'm going to tell you all about it in the hope that you will learn from it and not have to suffer for as long as I did. I want to help you break free of the dieting trap and shorten your learning curve, so you don't waste 25 years of your life like I did.

My deepest desire is for you to finally release yourself from your diet prison and go out and do what you were meant to do. For you to quit living such a small life, silencing your voice and killing your dreams while you stay stuck in your house on a diet.

Yes, I want to help you lose weight. But that's just the beginning. What I really want is to help you not only shed pounds and look and feel better, but to start setting and achieving meaningful goals — the long-forgotten goals you had as a girl — and live the life you should be living.

This book will show you how.

It's Not About the Weight

If I were given one hour to save the planet, I would spend 59 minutes defining the problem and one minute solving it.

— Albert Einstein

D o you remember the Jim Carrey movie *The Truman Show*? It was about a man whose whole life was a television show, created by a company that supplies actors who conspire to keep the fabricated existence going and keep him oblivious to reality.

The poor guy has no idea what's happening, because everyone's in on it. Gradually, however, he starts to see signs that something's not right, and he ultimately figures out that he's been living in a false world that he can actually escape from.

Now, change the main character from male to female, and multiply that character by hundreds of thousands of women.

You are one of those women. And so was I — until I figured out what was happening and escaped.

If I asked you what you would wish for if you could have anything, I'll bet you'd say to lose weight. If you could change one thing about your life, you'd say you'd want to be thin or to have the perfect body. But I'm going to tell you right now, with absolute certainty, that this isn't what you really want. Really, it's not.

What you really want is the *feeling* you'll have once you lose the weight. What you're after is the life you imagine living once the weight is gone.

This is a critical distinction, because once you make it, everything falls into place. That's because when you finally see that this feeling is what you're actually striving for, you can get busy working toward that life, rather than killing yourself trying to change the number on your scale.

And guess what? If you were already living that "thin life," you would automatically get the number you've been so desperate to see. And you wouldn't be having to spend your days praying that you have what it takes not to binge on chocolate or to have enough strength to make yourself order a salad instead of a cheeseburger.

The irony is that by wasting all your time forcing yourself to do these things, you're actually pushing that ideal life further and further away from you. Instead, what you should be doing is choosing to go ahead and live the life you dream of. Then you would naturally gravitate toward all the healthy behaviors — the ones you're currently forcing yourself to do — that would make you thin.

What you're doing now is living a half-lived life. I don't say that lightly, because I used to live that life, too. If you're focused exclusively on losing weight, your life isn't the joy-filled one you dream of — the one you should be living.

The problem with the half-lived life is that it automatically consists of habits that keep your body out of alignment with health. This life keeps the weight on your body. It makes your skin dull and lifeless. It makes you feel tired and worn out.

Then you feel desperate to eliminate these things. But unfortunately, the weight, the bad skin, and the exhaustion are only symptoms. But feeling desperate makes you search for quick-fix solutions like diets, expensive face creams, and medications — which are temporarily alleviating the symptoms but never solving the real problem.

However, none of these symptoms would exist if you were living not to fill some inner void but rather living a life where the void didn't exist in the first place. In other words, the life you imagine living when you finally lose the weight.

Women everywhere believe that our ultimate goal is to lose weight and that there's nothing abnormal about wasting our lives doing it. It's insane, and the fact that we don't question it is even more so.

We're imprisoned by the intense, never-ending, obsessive desire to lose weight. We spend our lives talking about how much weight we've gained, what size we are, how many calories we just ate, and how many calories we just burned. We talk about what diet we're on and how much weight we're trying to lose. We talk about how hard it is to lose weight and how "disgusting" we look.

It doesn't matter if you're a working professional or a stay-at-home mom. It doesn't matter if you're married or single, or whether you have children or you don't. Regardless of your age, your career path, your marital status, or where you live, it's likely (especially if you're reading this book) that you don't like the way you look and want to lose weight.

It's also highly likely that you've spent the better part of your life obsessing about this one thing to the exclusion of all else and that you feel like a failure that you haven't been able to do it.

I have friends who are intelligent and have successful careers, women with advanced degrees and impressive job titles, who talk about losing weight as if it's impossible to do. I have friends who are teachers and counselors who spend their days empathizing with others, helping them feel supported and understood, treating themselves as if they were worthless. I have friends who are stay-at-home moms, spending nearly every hour of their days taking care of their families, but who do hardly anything for themselves.

I have friends from all walks of life for whom being solution-oriented, regardless of what they do all day, is a requirement — all of them brainwashed into believing that losing weight is impossible and that spending their entire lives trying to do it is normal. Believing that their worth is tied to what they look like. And believing that no matter what they've accomplished outside of that, they're failures because they can't lose weight.

The reason this pains me so much is that I did this for years. I spent my days agonizing silently over how I looked and what I could do to get rid of the extra weight. I fantasized about what my life would be like when I looked a certain way, and I reserved all my hopes and dreams and plans for the future until that arbitrary day finally showed up. I put my whole life on hold without even realizing it, waiting to really live until I finally lost weight.

I was so focused on my weight and how I could lose it that I eventually stopped noticing how absorbed I was with it; it ultimately became a natural and normal part of my life. As a result, I spent more than 25 years locked in a prison of my own making, suffering unnecessarily, until I finally realized that I had the keys to freedom — I only had to unlock the door and walk out.

If you think that finally losing the weight and looking different will change your life, you're wrong. I know you think that if you lost the weight and had the perfect body, then you'd be happy, you'd finally love yourself, and everything would fall into place for you.

But it's actually the reverse: when you start understanding why you use food to fill an internal void, you can stop shaming yourself for your bad habits and start caring for yourself and your body. You can accept yourself exactly as you are and start developing healthy habits that make you feel good about yourself — and the results of which start to show up outwardly. You can take the confidence you generate from doing these things to set and achieve meaningful goals.

And once you do all of this, everything falls into place: your eating habits, your relationship with food, the way you think, the way you feel, the way you see yourself — and, yes, the body you live in.

So, the weight is there for a reason — it's just a symptom of a much bigger problem.

Weight is a symptom

We live in a culture that is obsessed with losing weight.

Walk past a rack of magazines at the grocery store, and nearly every one advertises a way for women to lose weight. Turn on the television, and you'll see an advertisement for the latest diet. Listen in on any conversation between women, and the topic of losing weight will inevitably come up.

It's pervasive. You can barely go a whole day without hearing about some new approach to get rid of the weight.

But if it's such an obsession with everyone, and there's such a constant, relentless focus on it — why haven't we all lost it? Wouldn't you think that by now someone would have finally solved the problem and can tell us how to do it?

There's a good reason why this hasn't happened. And the reason is that it's not about the weight.

We've been brainwashed into believing that the weight is the problem. And all the diet makers, exercise gurus, and nutrition specialists keep trying to persuade you that weight is your problem, that you should get rid of it, and that they are the only ones who can show you how.

The issue with this is that we can't see the forest for the trees. We keep running from one diet to the next — from the one that says carbs are the problem to the other that says too much fat is the issue.

We're so focused on the weight and trying to get rid of it that we can't see the bigger picture. And the bigger picture is that the weight isn't the problem. It's only a symptom of the problem.

The real problem is the way you eat. And you eat the way you do for specific reasons that only you can determine and that are unique to you and your experiences here on this planet.

Part of the issue is that you forget this, that there's a reason you eat the way you do — and it's not because you're lazy, weak-willed, or worthless. And the reason you haven't been able to lose it isn't because you don't have enough willpower or just can't stop eating.

But the whole time you're shaming yourself, the weight keeps showing up, again and again. And it will reliably continue to do so until you address the real problem.

Focusing on the weight keeps you from losing it

The first thing you need to know is that continuing to focus on the weight is the best possible way to keep yourself from ever losing it.

Sadly, this is extremely common, and our dieting culture perpetuates this. In fact, the entire dieting industry is built around having you focus exclusively on the weight — and hate it intensely enough that you will buy their product. (Maybe more than once.)

And because no diet will ever work long-term, regardless of what it requires you to do, all you're left with when it's over (in other words, when you "fail") is the weight.

The only reason you should ever focus on the weight is to objectively assess the situation so that you can build a plan to change it.

But we don't use any objectivity when it comes to weight. We attribute the weight to perceived personality or character defects. We're not persistent enough to stick to a diet. We don't have enough willpower to just stop eating. We're weak because we can't do it ourselves. We don't work out enough because we're lazy.

By focusing on the weight and jumping straight to the personal attack, you miss the opportunity to investigate and problem solve. Here's an example from my own life of a time when I got caught up in an emotional spiral because of not objectively figuring out what was going on, and I stayed stuck in it until I identified the real problem.

It used to make me really angry when I had no help around the house. I would seethe as I folded laundry and loaded the dishwasher. My anger was mostly directed toward my then-husband, because I obviously didn't expect my young children to help. Once everything was clean, my anger dissipated. But it always returned when I had to do it all over again without any help.

But instead of simply asking for help, I shamed myself for feeling angry. The critical voice in my head said things like, "What is the matter with you? Why are you getting so mad? Aren't you supposed to enjoy cleaning your home for your family? What kind of mother gets pissed off because she has to clean up after her children?"

I finally realized that I was only hurting myself by being angry, so instead I started asking myself better questions and giving myself honest answers. And those answers led me to even deeper questions.

Why does having no help make me so angry? Because I feel overloaded and no one notices. Why does it make me angry that no one notices? Because it makes me feel unappreciated. Why does feeling unappreciated upset me? Because it makes me feel like I'm not even here.

And then I finally figured out the real reason for my anger: feeling unappreciated and, therefore, disconnected.

It turns out my real problem was feeling disconnected. The symptom was the anger, but shaming myself for the anger kept me stuck being angry. I was so focused on the symptom (and judging myself for it) that I never solved the problem. It wasn't until I stepped back objectively, assessed the situation without judgment,

13

and asked myself constructive questions that I was able to get somewhere.

After that, whenever I felt a stab of rage every time my husband walked past me while I was breaking a sweat vacuuming, I stopped myself and remembered what was really going on. And I eventually was able to solve the problem by telling him I felt disconnected. Then we made a plan to find ways to feel more connected. It turned out that spending more quality time together made me feel less angry when I was doing chores by myself.

When you constantly focus on the symptom, feeling shame and judgment, instead of getting to the root of the problem with objectivity, you stay stuck. But when you solve the real problem, the symptoms take care of themselves.

One of the main reasons that staring at the weight, hating it, and judging yourself for it keeps you stuck is the resistance it creates. We'll talk more about this in the next chapter, but what happens is that resistance pushes you to do the very thing that you've trained yourself to do any time you feel it: eat. And eating in a disordered way keeps the weight on your body.

Figuring out how you trained yourself to eat the way you do is critical. It's the *why* that you need to figure out. Once you do this, you can address the real reasons and find solutions.

Focusing on what you look like will keep you far, far away from this process.

It's not what you eat, it's the way that you eat it

If you are going to address the problem instead of the symptom, it's vital to understand one very important thing: it's not what you eat — it's the way that you eat it.

This is a big reason diets don't work. Although none of them look the same, diets are all the same in one aspect. They focus on manipulating what you eat, rather than showing you how to change the way you eat.

Eat low-carb, eat high-carb, eat "clean" foods, eat for your blood type, go vegetarian. These are all different approaches that have the same variable: change what you eat until you get the result you're after.

Here is a possibly controversial and unpopular truth: what you eat is not as important as the way that you eat it. That's because until you change *how* you eat, what you eat is irrelevant.

I don't care if you're vegan, if you binge eat, you're not going to lose weight. Eating only clean foods (whatever that means) won't make you "clean" if you're scarfing them down in front of the television. Being a vegetarian for sure helps the planet — but not eating meat won't make you lose weight if you're shoving down everything on your plate.

When I was training for my first marathon in the late 90s, I experimented with eating different foods to see how they would affect my running. I gradually, without any intention of doing so, became a vegetarian.

However, even though I switched to a plant-based diet and was running anywhere from five to 20 miles a day, I didn't lose weight.

I remember clearly being at the end of my runs and thinking about all the food I was going to binge on because I "deserved it" and because the food was healthy.

I would get back from a long run, shower and dress, and head to a Mexican restaurant for a veggie burrito that could have easily fed four people. I inhaled the food in front of me, leaving the restaurant so full I almost felt sick.

Am I saying that it doesn't matter what your diet consists of? Of course not. But that's not what you should be worried about at first. Change how you eat, and the "what" part of it comes later.

No matter how many times you alter what you eat, nothing will change until you change how you eat. And furthermore, continuing to buy into the idea that you will somehow magically land on the perfect diet is a myth perpetuated to the extreme by the diet industry — and as long as you stay attached to this fantasy, you will never make progress.

So, remember: It's not what you eat, it's the way that you eat it.

Emotional eating

So, if it's the way that you eat that's the problem and you've been trying to lose weight for years and haven't been able to do it, it's almost certainly because you're an emotional eater.

We've all heard the term emotional eating, but what is it exactly? Well, it's exactly what it sounds like: eating in response to emotions.

If you eat emotionally, you eat because of how you feel emotionally rather than how you feel physically. You're eating in an emotional response to what's going on around you rather than eating in response to an objective, physical sensation caused by an extended lack of food. In other words, hunger.

But let's talk about hunger for a second. If you're an emotional eater, it's possible that you're never actually experiencing true hunger because of your habit of eating in response to environmental stimuli, which are ever present and frequently out of your control. It's also likely that you're attaching emotions to and making associations with the concept of hunger.

For example, if you feel hungry you may say, "I'm starving." Or you may associate time with being hungry: "I haven't eaten since lunch" or "It's dinner time" or "Breakfast is the most important meal of the day." And whether these things are or are not true, they are distracting you from objectively experiencing the feeling of hunger.

True hunger is capable of being endured for long periods of time — not that you should try to achieve this just so you can lose weight.

My point is, I'm pretty sure you have never been starving a day in your life. And just because it's noon doesn't necessarily mean it's time to eat.

The problem with assigning meanings and emotions to true, physical hunger is that you never see it objectively. As a result, you're making yourself incapable of making a conscious decision about what and when to eat. You're being reactive and grabbing whatever's in front of you, even if you're not truly hungry. And even if what's in front of you is good for you, if you eat emotionally, you're going to eat way too much of it to actually make it healthy.

So, how can you tell if you're an emotional eater? Here are some signs:

- You eat when you're not truly, physically hungry.
- You eat too fast.
- You eat past the point of fullness.
- You don't like eating in front of people or are embarrassed about how much you eat.
- The act of eating itself rather than the food you're eating is what's satisfying.

I think of eating emotionally as having an eating disorder. Just because you've never had what's traditionally considered an eating disorder, like bulimia or anorexia, you're still eating in a disordered way. And all that means is that you have an unhealthy relationship with food.

Emotional eating is also marked by other disordered behaviors like obsessing about what you eat, how much you should or shouldn't eat, and when you're going to eat next, and attaching feelings of shame and worthlessness to the act of eating.

How to stop eating emotionally

So how do you stop eating emotionally?

Obviously, it's taken you a lifetime to entrench these behaviors, so it's not going to go away overnight — if ever. That's because the triggers will always be there. What must change is how you respond to them.

I still have urges to binge eat and eat to make myself feel better. Those never go away. What's changed is that I act on them differently.

It takes reflection and inner work to figure this out. And I know your eyes are glazing over right now and that you just want to skip to the next chapter where I tell you exactly what to eat for the next ten days. (Spoiler: it's not going to happen.)

Believe it or not, time traveling back through your past can actually be fun. It only feels hard, because we've become conditioned to get an instant solution to a problem. In our convenience culture, you can program a destination a thousand miles away into your phone and it will lead you there automatically. So it feels painful to have to sit down, be quiet, think about our lives, and go through the messy work of figuring out on our own how to solve our problems.

Instead, think of it this way: imagine that you're sitting in a room by the fire with a bottle of wine with a trusted, compassionate friend who wants to do nothing else but hear you talk about yourself and your life. That's not so bad, is it?

The self-discovery process can not only be thoroughly enjoyable, but it's also the most important thing you'll ever do — because it's the foundation that sets you up to get the most success on your weight-loss journey.

And really, it's such a massive relief to figure out why you eat the way you do, because up until now all you've been doing is shaming yourself for it. But remember, you weren't born an emotional eater.

18

Eating emotionally is a learned behavior, and you taught yourself to do it to avoid pain. You didn't start eating emotionally because you love food so much or because you have no willpower or because you're out of control. You learned how to use eating as a bridge between pain and the absence of it.

Here's an exercise I used on myself to start my own healing process. (I highly recommend that you get a notebook out and write down your answers; your potential to get results multiplies exponentially just from the simple act of writing everything down.) There are two parts. First, answer these questions:

- What's the first time you remember using food to make yourself feel better?
- What did you eat, and what were you doing while you ate it?
- How did you feel after you ate? Satisfied, relived, ashamed, ugly, or worthless? (All of the above?)
- Did anyone make you feel ashamed of how much or what you ate? Who was it and what did they say?
- What patterns developed as a result of this event? Did you start eating alone in your room? Did you eat when no one was home? Did you develop certain cravings that you still have now?

I can remember vividly my first episodes of eating emotionally. I made things like bagels with cream cheese, biscuits drowning in butter, and French fries with ranch dressing. I would wait until no one was around and make a huge plate of one of these things, then lock myself in my parents' den and scarf everything down while I watched television.

I had the sense that I was doing something "wrong" or that I should be embarrassed about, and I felt ashamed of my behavior. I tried to hide, because if anyone saw me, they said things that made me feel like there was something wrong with me or that I couldn't control myself. (They did not do this intentionally or to be unkind; this is just how I internalized it.)

While I was eating it was like I was in a trance. I didn't just feel satisfied — I felt like I was high. And there was no question of stopping when I was full. I kept eating until there was nothing left. Also, it felt like nothing else in the world was happening — it was like an out-of-body experience. And watching television while I binged kept me zoned out even more.

After I ate, I was deeply ashamed of my behavior. I hated how stuffed I was and how out of control I felt. I got rid of the evidence as fast as I could so no one saw it and so they couldn't judge me. Most of all I judged myself for not being able to stop.

Okay, now here is the second, even more important part of the exercise. Figure out what drove you to eat in the ways you just described. Ask yourself these questions:

- How did you feel as a child growing up in your house?
- Who was the dominant figure in your household? Your mom? Your dad? Your older brother?
- How did that person behave? Were they constantly irritated? Was that person a good listener? Were they always gone? Were they always laughing? Were they passive? Aggressive? Sarcastic?
- How did their behaviors spill over into their relationship with you? Were they impatient with you? Did they make fun of you, even in a good-natured way? Did you feel anxious? Eager to prove yourself? Intent on not rocking the boat? How did they express their love to you?
- If you had to describe how you felt growing up in one word, what would it be?

- Most importantly, can you connect that feeling to learning how to eat to make yourself feel better or to make that feeling go away?

Here's how I answered those questions. My father was the dominant figure in my home, and he was an extreme workaholic. He wasn't gone a lot, but I still felt disconnected from him. Even though he was physically present, I felt like I was invisible to him because he was so busy working.

On top of that, my parents entertained frequently because of my father's job. I watched my father be super engaged with all the people that came through our house and internalized the message that there must be something wrong with me that he didn't interact with me the same way.

I have to give my disclaimer here — especially because he may be reading this! — that my father is one of the most generous, kind-hearted people I know, and he has done more to help other people than he ever has for himself. And he worked as hard as he did to give his family the kind of life he didn't have growing up.

The point of this exercise isn't to blame anyone or anything or to be a victim. My feelings growing up had nothing to do with what was or wasn't really happening — they were all a result of my interpretation of what was going on around me. And my interpretation is what caused some of my behaviors.

When you're an adult, you have the perspective to choose how you want to interpret the world around you. But when you're a child you merely react to your environment until you figure out what feels good or doesn't. And when you feel pain and you find something that makes it go away, you keep doing that thing — until it eventually becomes habitual.

So, the one word I would choose to describe how I felt growing up is . . . alone. Obviously, the food I ate wasn't actually going to make me feel less alone, but eating it make my feelings of isolation, loneliness, and being invisible temporarily go away. So, I kept doing it until eating became my go-to activity to feel better in any situation.

Later on, I lived alone in my own apartment by choice, so feeling "lonely" was no longer an issue for me. But stress and boredom were. And regardless of how extreme those sensations were — ranging anywhere from moderately uncomfortable to severely painful — I ate to make them go away, because that's what I had trained myself to do.

All of this boils down to understanding why you eat emotionally. Because once you understand that there's a reason for it and you figure out what it is, the judgment goes away. And when the judgment goes away, the shame goes with it.

Stop feeling ashamed

I think a lot of women, me included at one point, feel tremendous shame about the weight they see. They see the excess weight as an indicator of what kind of person they are — and not in a good way.

Sadly, our culture reinforces the concept that how you look determines your worth and if you don't look a certain, accepted way, you aren't worthy — and the more you deviate from the norm, the more worthless you are.

I used to see my weight as evidence that I was out of control, weak, and had no willpower. I was giving myself all kinds of labels and unnecessarily attaching emotions to the situation, when what I should have been doing was looking at it objectively.

It wasn't until about age 35 that I finally figured this out. And just because I did doesn't mean that I don't ever run into some slip-ups and "failures" in my own life.

For example, a few years ago I went through an extremely difficult time in my life. Over the course of a year, my marriage deteriorated until it ultimately ended in divorce.

22

The fighting, the anger, and the chaos triggered my emotional eating, and it came back full force. I hate to say it, but I binge ate (and drank) and hardly worked out. Over the course of six months, I gained ten pounds.

Of course, I wasn't happy about it. I was emotionally drained, and it showed up on the outside. But instead of hating my body and being ashamed of the way I looked, I knew from experience that I had no choice but to embrace it.

It wasn't easy, but I made a conscious decision to not feel bad about falling off the wagon so completely. I realized that the weight got there because of how I coped with the trauma I went through — and that was to eat emotionally because of my deep-seated association between eating and feeling better I developed as a child.

So, even though I wasn't happy about the weight, I decided to embrace it — and carry it proudly. I decided that, rather than being a badge of shame, it was actually a symbol of strength. Because it represented the fact that I went through the worst time in my life, and I came out of it on the other side — stronger, better. And that's beautiful.

If you want to make changes in your life, including losing weight, shame must be eliminated. That's because shame equals paralysis. Shame prevents you from taking action and keeps you from growing. As long as you allow shame to be part of the equation, you will never make permanent changes — or any changes at all.

Shame keeps you stuck, because it keeps you in an emotionally driven mindset. Anytime you introduce emotions into a scenario, you can't see anything objectively. If you have a disagreement with someone that makes you feel angry, you can't see anything clearly and possibly apologize and make amends (or decide you're not going to put up with their behavior and walk away entirely). If you feel afraid of doing something, staying stuck in that fearful place won't allow you to make a plan to take control of the situation and feel less afraid of doing it. Keeping yourself in an emotionally charged place prevents you from seeing clearly and taking constructive action.

Even worse, shame makes you feel "less than." It creates the false belief that everyone in the world is actively judging you. And there's nothing more disempowering than that.

When you listen to your inner critic (more on that later), the louder that mean-girl voice in your head gets. And although you can't completely get rid of it, you can at least turn down the volume.

The first way to do this is to recognize that the voice isn't real and that what it's saying is false. Feeling judged by other people is human, but realize that people are generally far too worried about what they look like to spend time worrying about what you look like.

The next thing you have to do is embrace everything about yourself — including the weight. You have to learn to love what you see. It's actually not that hard to do once you take to heart everything I've said in this chapter. Ultimately, the weight is there because of some sort of pain you experienced long ago. You had to use something to cope, and for you it was food. There is nothing wrong with it, and it's certainly nothing to be ashamed of. And the longer you keep feeling ashamed of it, the longer the weight will stay there.

Excess weight has nothing to do with who you are. It's an indicator, nothing more. It's a sign that you're merely taking the wrong actions in the wrong way. (And if you're trying to diet it off, you're doing *everything* wrong.)

The very good news is that it's really easy to fix your approach. But you're just delaying it as long as you allow yourself to feel shame.

It feels hard to overcome shame, especially when our whole culture promotes the idea that what we as women look like is of the utmost importance. But once you decide to override the feeling of shame by choosing to face what you currently see in the mirror and embrace it because of understanding where it came from, then you can make a plan and take action to change it.

As Brené Brown says, "Shame corrodes the very part of us that believes we are capable of change."

Remember, the weight is there for a reason. (And it's not because of who you are.) It's just a sign that you need to do things differently. And it's almost impossible to convince yourself that you're capable of making changes when you're busy giving yourself the constant message that you're worthless and powerless. You're anything but, and this problem is completely solvable.

Seeing the weight as a symptom rather than the actual problem takes the emotion out of it and allows you to see things clearly. And, as I'm about to tell you, there are unlimited changes you can make to get things moving and start making progress.

Once you understand that it's how you eat and not what you eat that's the issue, you can change it. As long as you keep yourself in the forest, chasing one path (diet) after the next, hoping that it will lead you out, you'll stay stuck, blindly roaming the forest — with an evil voice in the background telling you how pathetic you are for not being able to find your way out.

The only thing you've been missing is a map. And the map is different for every person. That's because you have to create your own, which is what I'll show you how to do. Your map is different from mine because you live a totally different life than I do. Your map doesn't look like your best friend's map, because her motivations for eating emotionally aren't the same as yours.

The process of designing and using your own map means you're taking responsibility for yourself and putting yourself in a place of power and control over your own results — both the ones you've gotten up until now and the ones you'll see in the future. By creating your own plan you'll no longer keep yourself in a place of powerlessness where you think your only option is for a diet to tell you what to do. You'll rip yourself out of the mindset that there's a winning lottery ticket that will fix everything.

You are not powerless, it's not that complicated, you can handle it, and you can do it.

Not only that, you'll be so busy simultaneously designing an exciting, goal-centered life for yourself that you'll be too busy and too energized to sit around thinking about what you're not supposed to eat.

Resistance

Whatever you fight you strengthen,
and what you resist persists.

— *Eckhart Tolle*

If you've been trying to lose weight for years, the feeling of resistance should be very familiar to you.

You feel it when you look at your body, when you try not to eat certain foods, and when you force yourself to work out. Actually, your primary goal is resistance-backed: *lose* weight.

And the thing is, we're all so used to the resistance of the whole endeavor that we expect it. Losing weight is hard, right?

This is a critical point: the resistance inherent in dieting and the resistance that we expect to encounter when trying to lose weight is what actually makes it so hard to lose it — and it's what ultimately keeps us from losing it.

Feeling resistance of any kind keeps you away from whatever it is you're trying to achieve. It's an unnecessary hurdle you're inserting in your path that you have to jump over on your way to your goal. Feeling resistant essentially means that you're working against yourself.

First of all, what is resistance? According to Merriam-Webster, resistance is "the act of exerting force in opposition of something." Let's look at that carefully.

The first word that stands out is *opposition*, meaning that whatever action you're taking, you're going against something — you're exerting energy to oppose it. The second key word is *force*, meaning you're working really hard to oppose whatever it is you're resisting.

But an interesting thing happens when you do this. Whatever you're pushing back on will meet you with the same push back. If you remember Newton's third law of physics: For every action, there is an equal and opposite reaction. Not only that, to the extent that you oppose something, that thing will meet you with the same force and intensity.

The point I'm making is obvious, I hope. The more you resist something, the more difficult it will be to make it not happen. Therefore, the more you resist the weight, the harder it is to get rid of.

It's counterintuitive, but in order to lose weight, you have to stop fighting against it. Instead, you have to embrace it.

How it keeps you stuck

This quote by Mother Teresa perfectly sums up how resistance stops you from achieving what you want: "I will never attend an anti-war rally, but if you have a peace rally, invite me."

She knew that working toward peace was far more effective than fighting against war, because fighting against war in an effort to create more peace actually pushes peace away. The energy you stir up in opposition to a war is the antithesis of peace.

If you fight against anything, you create more of it. And I know you've seen this in your own life.

For example, we all have that friend who loves to spout off her opinions on just about every subject and is practically challenging you to a debate. The friend with a bag full of polarizing conversation topics, ready to launch out into the cocktail party to see who's up for an argument.

You know from experience that the absolute worst thing you can do if you want to end a conversation with a person like this is to fight her. Instead, you simply mumble a few mmm-hmm's and say "I know what you mean" as many times as it takes to satisfy her. You know that if you push back on her, you're going to get the same, or even stronger, push back. And it will never end until you stop resisting her and let her go her own way.

Another example is what lifeguards always teach you. If you find yourself suddenly struggling in the ocean, do not swim against the tide — go with the current. (There are even signs on the beach with a little diagram that shows you how to do it.)

If you argue with your friend, you'll stay stuck in the pointless, one-sided argument. If you fight the waves, you're going to drown. And if you try to lose the weight, you're never going to lose it.

Trying to lose weight practically ensures that you won't. And that's just the "opposition" part — don't forget about the "force" part. Trying to get rid of it will keep it there, and the more intensely you focus on it and fan the internal flames of disgust and hatred, the more difficult it will be to lose it.

So what's the single best way to make sure you don't lose weight? Go on a diet.

How dieting makes it worse

You walk right into the lion's den of failure when you go on a diet. In fact, you couldn't devise a more effective way to fail.

To make sure you buy what they're selling, the diet makers have to make you focus exclusively on the weight and hate it intensely enough to believe that their program is the only one that works. They have to build your antagonism and disgust to the point that you'll pay anything for the magic bullet they're serving up to you on a silver platter.

It's also in the diet makers' best interest to cultivate a feeling of failure on your part so that you feel even more desperate. Part of their hook is that you've dieted and failed so many times that you feel a sense of urgency and desperation to go on this one special diet that is the answer to your problem and that will finally change your life.

So, they all keep selling you the same flawed product, dressed up in different ways, that promises you the miracle. But none of them — no matter how different they seem on the surface — will ever work because of one simple fact: they're all about resistance.

And the worst part of all is that because you've been so brainwashed into believing that this is the one diet that absolutely works, when it doesn't, *you* are the failure. And your confidence is now even lower that it was, and you're that much more susceptible to the next false promise from yet another diet maker.

And, of course, it doesn't work the next time, and you stay stuck in the dieting downward spiral.

We'll get to the specifics of why diets never work in the next chapter. But the primary reason none of them do is because of the resistance they create.

Types of resistance

A key element of resistance is that it eventually has to be neutralized. Feeling resistant, quite simply, doesn't feel good.

Any time you feel resistance, you will eventually do something to counterbalance it. If you're running up the final hill of a 5K, you're anticipating the other side of where you will coast back down. If you've been pushing yourself all day to get everything done, you're going to unwind at the end of it with a glass of wine or a few hours of Netflix. And if you work really hard not to eat anything, you're eventually going to give in and binge.

It's worse when it comes to dieting, because the thing you're resisting (eating) is the very thing you've trained yourself to do to make yourself feel better. So, going for hours without eating will result in a major binge for someone who's an emotional eater.

But whereas a Netflix binge won't sabotage your health or drain your confidence — at worst, you'll only have wasted a few hours of your day — binge eating not only wrecks your health, it also drains your confidence. And because you stay locked in this diet/fail/binge cycle, your confidence erodes to the point you lose faith in yourself altogether.

You can't feel resistance for too long before you need relief from it. And the longer you try to sustain it, the more intense your desire will be to neutralize it. In other words, the longer you diet, the more your desire to binge will intensify and the more often you'll do it.

There are two types of resistance that come with dieting and trying to lose weight. Let's look at those.

Resistance toward your body

The most obvious kind of resistance that comes with trying to lose weight is your resistance toward your body. It feels completely normal for you to resist your own body, because we've all been so conditioned to do it that it's practically a social pastime.

I don't know if I've ever been to a girls' night out, had a phone conversation with a friend, or even watched some kind of television show geared toward women where there wasn't some sort of reference to how we look and what we want to change about ourselves. It's to the point that we no longer see ourselves as whole human beings but rather a collection of body parts.

You may not be fully aware of this, but think about how many times you talk about yourself in terms of parts of your body. Like

31

how much you hate your stomach or your jiggly arms or your boobs that now sag after breastfeeding your babies (how sad).

Thinking of yourself in terms of body parts reinforces resistance to your body. That's because if you're constantly mentally cutting yourself apart like this, you're far less likely to consider the things that are beautiful and that make you "whole." You're also far less likely to develop eating habits based on health and far more likely to take drastic measures and eat in a disordered way. If you want to feel more vibrant and alive, it's easy to increase your desire to eat as many fruits and vegetables as you can. If you want to get rid of your muffin top, you'll be motivated to crash diet or try not to eat.

It took me a very, very long time to stop thinking of myself this way — or even to notice that I was doing it at all. I mean, all my friends talked about themselves the same way, and other people even pointed out what parts of me they thought didn't measure up. And, unfortunately, I listened to them.

Case in point: several years ago, I was on a date, and I had my really heavy purse slung over my shoulder. My arm was pressed up against my side, and the skin on my inner arm had gotten pinched up under the strap of my purse. I was happily chatting away when all of a sudden, my date said, "Someone needs to work on her arms a little bit."

I stopped mid-sentence and felt embarrassment and shame wash over me. In that moment I was reduced to a body part — one that was unattractive (at least to him) and clearly unacceptable.

Rather than tell him to go eff himself — which is what I should have done and exactly what I would do now — I let his words rip a hole through my self-esteem and in that instant change how I saw myself. It's sad to say, but I remember those words every single time I put on a sleeveless shirt or throw my purse over my shoulder.

Before that incident, I had never given my arms a thought. After it, I added my arms to my mental list of body parts I didn't like. And this mental list of perceived distortions continued to compel me to diet myself to perfection and to eat accordingly.

The media reinforces this disconnection with our bodies. This is a well-known phenomenon by now, but it's worth repeating. And even if you think you're immune, know that on a subconscious level we are all deeply affected by it.

However, resistance to our bodies isn't limited to the mental realm. It also manifests physically.

Doing things like sucking in your stomach to look skinner, pressing your arms out so they don't look big, or crossing your legs so your cellulite doesn't show creates physical resistance. If inner resistance is draining, the physical resistance caused by all these contortions is flat-out crippling.

Think of how often you do this throughout the day. It feels miserable to stand in all these awkward positions — and not only that, it reinforces the mental resistance you have because it focuses all your attention squarely on your body and what you don't like about it.

On a deeper level, it also puts all your energy on you, which disconnects you from everyone and everything around you. And if you aren't connected with others, you aren't really living.

How often do you walk confidently into a room without worrying about how other people are perceiving you in that moment? Or how often do you listen intently to what someone else is saying rather than waiting to chime in or mentally reviewing what you just said, wondering if you sounded stupid?

Our looks-focused, prestige-driven culture makes connecting with other people next to impossible because it makes us focus exclusively on ourselves and wondering how we're coming across. And this relentless focus on ourselves and attempting to be anything less than hilariously funny, super impressive, and flawless looking is confidence-draining and exhausting — which, ironically, means we end up being none of those things.

Here's another way to look at it: think about how little girls carry themselves and how they interact with each other.

When I watch my daughters play together, they are utterly *un*-self-conscious (in the most literal sense). They are fully engaged in all their moments and have yet to become hyper-focused on their looks. The last thing they're doing when they're running, playing, or simply standing still is worrying about what they look like.

They haven't developed the habits I mentioned earlier — of sucking everything in or hiding behind a piece of furniture so no one sees how "fat" they are. They don't avoid having their picture taken because they look "disgusting." Actually, they can't have their photograph taken often enough. (It's actually me that's usually trying to get out of the picture . . . is there anything more horrifying than an accidental selfie? See, I still struggle.)

It's beautiful to watch, and it reminds me of how sad it is that we as women obsess about how we look, hate and resist our bodies, and try to hide ourselves so much. It's beautiful not only because I'm their mom but also because I know intimately what it's like to do the opposite. (I sucked my stomach in for so long I'm surprised I didn't burn enough calories to get rid of it.)

Attempting to shrink yourself physically results in a shrunken life. And dieting and trying to lose weight is the perfect activity for someone who isn't really living. Again, that's what this whole book is ultimately about — me trying to get you to see how small you're living and helping you to escape this painful trap and go out into the world and really live.

Resisting your body means that you'll never take up your space. You'll keep getting out of everyone else's way, staying quiet and not saying what you need to say, apologizing when no apology is required. You'll spend your whole life pleasing everyone but yourself.

As long as you keep resisting your body, you'll keep trying to fix it to make it acceptable. And as long as you're dieting, you're going to keep resisting your body because dieting only reinforces the dissatisfaction that you feel toward it. So, you'll stay stuck for a lifetime: hating your body, dieting to fix it, failing, blaming yourself for the failure, hating yourself even more — and eating to make it all better.

Resistance toward food

The second type of resistance that goes with dieting is resistance toward food. Honestly, we have a seriously messed up attitude toward food in our culture — and not just when it comes to dieting.

Our balls-to-the wall, 24-7, achievement-driven culture does nothing to promote a healthy attitude toward eating. It's actually in direct opposition to it.

Food is meant to be enjoyed. And there's nothing enjoyable about inhaling a hamburger and fries at your desk while you're working, eating so fast you can hardly breathe. Or shoving some of your kids' fries down while you drive everyone to dance class and then hating yourself later.

Have you ever been to Europe? Europeans have a much healthier attitude toward food and eating. They spend a few hours at a meal, leisurely eating several small courses while enjoying conversation with whomever they're eating. The meal might be served with a bottle of good wine, which is slowly enjoyed by the participants (not just one of them).

When I lived in France, I worked at the front desk of a small hotel. Lunch was served every day from 12:00 until 3:00. We walked down the street to a restaurant, ordered and enjoyed a three- or four-course meal with a bottle of red wine, and headed back to the hotel around 2:00. The extra hour of the lunch break was reserved for — can you believe it? — napping.

Contrast that with what we do in America. We order one huge course that is scarfed down in record time, but not before whipping out our credit card for the server before he's even taken the plate. Check please!

We eat too fast, we eat too much, and we don't enjoy what we eat. Then when it's over, we're overstuffed and ready for that European nap — except for us it's more like a food coma. And we can't take it anyway, because it's time to get back to work.

Because of this distorted approach to food and eating, we have no concept of what true hunger is, how to properly respond to it, and how to develop eating habits based on its cues. And this unhealthy attitude toward eating fuels a fear of food.

But there's nothing good or bad about food. It's the mindset that we've adopted toward it that creates the concept that it's is something to be feared or avoided or that we're not "supposed" to eat.

If we looked at food objectively, we would take all the emotion out of it. But we don't do this. Instead, we set food up as this magnetic force that's luring us toward it and that we have to use all of our willpower to resist. But think about how crazy this is. There's nothing powerful or sinister about a plate of pasta. You can eat it . . . or not.

Setting food up this way gives it power over you. Food has no power, and it certainly isn't something that should control the way you live and dominate your every thought, dictating what you do all day.

Food is really no big deal. We give it more weight (pardon the pun) than it deserves. It has no more power than the chair you're sitting in or the coffee you drink or the car you drive. It just is. But the way you look at it — the way you obsess about it and fuel an abnormal fear of it — is a very big deal. Fear of food is a huge part of the problem and what needs to change.

Dieting reinforces this fear. In fact, diets are predicated on the fear of some type of food or food group. Carbs are evil, inflammatory foods are poisonous, saturated fat will kill you. And whether these foods are good for you or not — in fact, too much saturated fat isn't good for you and foods loaded with high-fructose corn syrup aren't healthy — none of these things are anything to be afraid of. The fact is, you won't buy a diet if whoever made it doesn't create some sort of irrational fear in your mind first.

What happens when you set up food as something to be afraid of is this: You avoid it like the plague and, in doing so, make it highly desirable. You've created resistance toward it, which has to be neutralized, and because you've trained yourself to eat to feel better, that is what you'll do — only now you have the forbidden food set up on a mental silver platter, ready for you to give in to.

A fearful attitude toward food leads to eating disorders, anorexia in one extreme and binge eating in the other. And somewhere in the middle is you: scared of certain foods, avoiding them, eventually bingeing on them, and starting all over. And the whole time it was never the food — it was you and your perception of it.

One positive thing about our relentless focus on food is that we know which ones nourish our bodies the most. Fruits, vegetables, whole grains, and nuts and seeds, to name a few. And we all know the benefits of drinking pure water. It's a good thing to be aware of what foods contain the most nutrients and that promote health and to be aware of those that, over time, don't.

But keep in mind that not only are foods not the enemy, they aren't the miracle either. And it's this type of extreme thinking and these kinds of radical attitudes that keep fueling our collective fear of food.

Actually, we're almost too aware of what the healthy foods are, to the point of being totally preoccupied with them. We're overly concerned with how much selenium a Brazil nut has and how deficient we are in that one nutrient. And, once again, we miss the forest for the trees.

Vitamins and minerals, and the names we have for them, are concepts. We've named these nutrients, and we have a useful system for categorizing them. But think of all the nutrients that are yet to be "discovered" and named by us.

There are potentially hundreds of thousands of substances hidden in all the healthy foods we eat, and they all work together to make that food support the proper functioning of our bodies. That is why it makes sense to eat the foods that are obviously healthy without trying to figure out how many grams of this or that are in them. (Basically, if you go to the store and spend most of your time in the produce section, you'll be okay. Simple.)

Not only that, but we've become almost totally disconnected from eating real food. We're so intent on not getting too many fat grams or focused on cutting calories that we've warped our interpretation of what food actually is.

Subsisting on Lean Cuisines is about as far away from what eating should look like that it's mind-blowing. We're so used to eating food that barely resembles its starting point that it seems normal. We buy food that initially came out of the ground, but it's gone through at least twenty steps before it gets to our plate.

If you eat a frozen diet meal of chicken parmigiana with broccoli, it may have started as a chicken on a farm (probably not, but that's another topic for another book) and a stalk of broccoli. But then what happens?

The food sits for a few days and is then processed and treated with chemicals to give it color and preserve its freshness. Then it's placed in a plastic container with cellophane and frozen and stored until it's time to pack it on a truck, where it travels cross-country for a few days. Then it sits in your grocery store's freezer for a few weeks until you buy it. Then you stick it in your freezer for another week, until you scarf it and its 300 calories down — yay, it's healthy! — for a truly unsatisfying "meal."

There is nothing physically healthy about eating food like this, and there's nothing mentally healthy about thinking that eating this way is normal.

Besides the issue of what is healthy or unhealthy, we totally miss out on the concept of food as enjoyment. And not only that, we hardly ever consider the process of cooking as enjoyable, energizing, and a creative experience — instead we look at it as a hassle, something we don't feel like doing, and a chore that's to be avoided at all costs.

Eating, if done properly, can be pleasurable. If you eat slowly and create a relaxing environment to eat in, eating becomes an experience — rather than a free-for-all, where you pay no attention to what you're actually eating while you shove it down.

Taking your time to conceive of, prepare, and eat a delicious meal takes every shred of fear out of the equation. Even if you make something less-than-healthy, if you plan it, take the time to make it, and eat it slowly and consciously, you're going to enjoy it and appreciate it more because you prepared it, and you're certainly not going to disrespect all your efforts by annihilating it in five minutes or less. And on some inexplicable, spiritual level that I can't explain, the food nourishes you more if it's eaten this way. I can't prove this of course, but I believe it's true.

How do you get rid of your fear of food? You don't completely get rid of it — at least not at first. It takes practice.

Getting rid of resistance

Eliminating resistance toward your body

This process is ultimately about you loving your body just the way it is now and accepting yourself, weight and all. But it's not enough for me to simply tell you this — you have to embrace this shift in mindset. Your resistance toward your body may be too entrenched a feeling to simply switch from one way of thinking to the other. You also need concrete actions that will get you from Point A to Point B.

I'm about to give you some of those actions, but first consider something that most people never do. It's a powerful concept to absorb that will get you over the hurdle.

The reason almost no one considers it is the attitude of failure we adopt toward ourselves. We're incredibly harsh on ourselves whenever we stumble and fall — and we tend to think of all of our stumbles as failures. Worse, we come to believe that we're the failures.

But think about it this way: It has taken you a lifetime to get the body you have and see every day. That body has been through good times and bad times — happy experiences and horrible moments, euphoria and trauma, passion and pain. You haven't arrived at the physical state you're in simply because you binge ate potato chips and didn't work out enough.

And to reiterate, emotional eating evolves in an effort to cope with some sort of pain you experienced early on. It's a huge relief to finally get this. That's because this knowledge helps you stop blaming your current eating behaviors on the idea that you have no self-control or that there's something wrong with you.

Although it's imperative that you take responsibility for where you are, responsibility doesn't involve either making excuses for your bad habits (I don't have time, being overweight runs in my family) or shaming yourself for having them. A person who is stuck in either of these places is incapable of taking responsibility, so both of these attitudes have to go if you want to make real changes. You have to accept and take responsibility for where you are if you want to go somewhere different.

Seeing yourself as a strong, resilient person who has come through all kinds of struggles (that are legitimate no matter what they are because they are real to you) is a beautiful thing. You're still here, and you're accomplishing a lot more than you give yourself credit for.

It's no small thing to take care of not only yourself but other people, too. Even if you don't have kids, you may be looking after your parents or being a support system to friends who are struggling. And even if you're not doing those things, working a full-time job doesn't leave a lot of energy for the self-care that we women are so used to ignoring but that is so desperately needed.

So, if you think about it, your body is basically a physical manifestation of all of your life experiences — and it can't be any other way. Really, it is what it is, and you have two choices: accept it or keep fighting it. If you accept it, even though you may not like it, you've taken the first step toward changing it. But if you keep fighting it, you'll stay stuck right where you are.

Okay, now that you've gotten a new perspective on all this, let's look at some specific things you can do to start releasing the resistance you have toward your body. There are two primary things you do day-to-day to resist your body: 1) listen to your inner critic, and 2) constrict your body. I'll address the inner critic in a later chapter, so let's discuss in more detail how constricting your body creates massive resistance.

You're probably so used to contorting your body into all kinds of uncomfortable positions that the resistance you feel has become a natural state. Doing things like sucking in your stomach and twisting yourself sideways in your chair so no one can see the cellulite on your legs is hugely resistant and miserable to feel. And I know this intimately from years of personal experience.

Sidebar: I'm going to talk here just about the physical resistance we create, but don't forget that there's an emotional toll that comes with doing things like avoiding having your picture taken, not showing up for a party because you think you look fat, and wrapping your towel around you at the pool just to walk two feet to get your sunscreen. These are things you can and should work on, but they will become much easier to overcome once you start relaxing into your body with the simple exercises I'm about to give you.

They seem simple or even ridiculous at first, because you're not truly aware of how often you resist your own body. But once you start practicing these exercises, you will quickly realize how often you constrict your body because of how foreign it will feel to finally relax.

1. Don't suck it in. Your energy begins in the center of your body, so if you're constricting yourself from the middle, what you're doing is negating all of your emotions and feelings.

It sounds woo-woo, but if you're holding yourself in physically, you're literally shoving down everything you feel. If you don't express your feelings, especially anger and pain, you turn them on yourself and engage in self-destructive behaviors, like binge eating.

While you're in the privacy of your own home, deliberately and consciously don't suck your stomach in. Walk around naturally and comfortably, move more slowly, breathe more deeply.

Notice how releasing this resistance changes how you think. Notice how the negative voice in your head starts to dissipate and a more compassionate voice emerges. Notice what a relief it is to finally let it all hang out. Once you get used to doing this, you can practice doing it more outside of your house.

2. Loosen up. Take off your skinny jeans and wear something comfortable once in a while! It's tempting to feel like wearing something really tight to help hold everything in is a good thing, but really it just creates more resistance.

Having to adjust your underwear that's wedged all up in there because your pants are so tight, and constantly pulling your waistband over your muffin top every time you stand up is exhausting and the opposite of relaxing into your body.

You don't have to slouch around in sweatpants and a ratty old t-shirt, but try wearing clothes that are a little less constricting. You can still be stylish and buy the same high-end brand you like — but maybe just stop ordering them one size too small.

Wearing clothes that aren't so tight or fitted really helps you take the focus off your body and makes it a lot easier to also practice not holding it in all the time. And it also feels good to be able to take a deep breath.

3. Look up. Worrying constantly about what you look like keeps you looking down, staring at your body and obsessing about it, instead of looking at what's out there in front of you — especially the people you're supposedly connecting with. When you constantly look down, you're not only constricting your body, you're narrowing your perspective overall.

Look up instead. Look at what's going on around you. Just looking up and out helps you hold yourself differently — you'll stand taller and take up your space more, both of which make you feel more powerful and confident. And it's a lot easier to let your body relax when you're not staring at it constantly, wondering if everyone else thinks you look fat.

While you're adopting these three simple practices, try to fully realize the mental benefits of letting your body go like this. Make mental notes — or even better, actual notes in a journal — of how your thoughts, feelings, and actions change as a result. Do you feel more peaceful and less critical of yourself? Do you have less of a desire to binge? Do you feel more relaxed around food and less fearful of it? Do you feel like you have more creative energy?

Creative energy is amazing, because you can use it to your advantage. Try something new. Eat at a new restaurant, go shopping for something you don't usually wear (hopefully, less form-fitting), get a massage. Taking yourself out of your rut and building on the good feelings you have spills over into all areas of your life, most importantly how you eat.

It's so much easier to make healthy choices when you're not working against yourself physically. Doing these exercises and making these mental shifts helps you love your body instead of hating it — which makes you want to take care of it instead of beating it into submission.

Eliminating resistance toward food

The main goal in eliminating your resistance toward food is to make it work for you rather than you working against it.

Instead of constantly fighting food and being afraid of it, you have to make peace with it and use it to your benefit. To do this, you have to do three things: 1) see food for what it is, 2) allow yourself to eat all kinds of foods, 3) and learn to enjoy the food you eat.

The dieting mentality makes you afraid of food and keeps you trying to be in control around it. It gives food power over you.

But again, food has no power. None. You're the one with the power. You have a choice to eat something or not eat it — or even to choose not to eat it for the rest of your life. But you can't make choices when you're putting yourself in a position of powerlessness. Making choices and decisions means you are in control — and you are.

So, making food something that you have to fight or try to avoid is not only absurd, it's disempowering. And you have to empower yourself (or rather, reclaim the power you've had all along) if you want to make real changes in your life.

Here are some strategies to change how you see and use food:

1. Eat based on how you feel. By this I don't mean eat a family-sized bag of chips because you feel like it. What I mean is, how do you actually *feel*? Are you truly hungry?

All too often, we eat based on environmental cues. We eat when we think it's time to eat. We eat because we're on our lunch break. We eat because we're out for dinner, even though we just ate a huge snack an hour ago. We eat because it's time for breakfast, we eat because we haven't eaten since breakfast. We don't allow ourselves to feel true hunger.

If you're not capable of identifying what true hunger is, you also won't be able to identify what foods you need most at what times — a practice that helps you make healthier choices.

For example, thinking you're hungry may simply mean you are dehydrated. Obviously, feeling thirsty means you should drink water, but there are also tons of foods that not only hydrate you, they give you valuable nutrients.

I can immediately tell if I'm hungry or if I'm dehydrated. I've practiced this often enough to spot the difference. Because of this, I now crave oranges or cucumbers instead of chips or a bagel with cream cheese. I know that the latter two won't satisfy me, and my body will keep looking for what it needs until I provide it.

You have to stop and assess what you're really feeling. Are you truly hungry or is it just "time" to eat? Taking even just a few moments to consider this is an act of control that gives you confidence.

2. Change your language. Oh, my Lord, the things we say when it comes to food. And these things are what create food's perceived power over us. "A moment on the lips, a lifetime on the hips," "Food is not your friend," "I'm a chocoholic," "I'm obsessed with French fries." Sound familiar?

You have to use more moderate language. First of all, enough with the cutesy sayings. If you've seen it in a sarcastic meme on Instagram, it's guaranteed you shouldn't say it. Food definitely isn't your "friend" — it's just food.

Instead of being a chocoholic, say what you really mean. Say that you really enjoy chocolate and like ending your meal with a piece of chocolate or a bite of a chocolate dessert. Instead of being obsessed with fries, keep it real. Say that you *like* French fries — and have some every once in a while.

Practice moderation in your language, and you'll easily be able to practice moderation when you eat.

3. Slow down. Eating too fast has many drawbacks. It means you're going to eat more than you need to, which equals weight gain. It means you never really enjoy the food you eat or the experience of eating itself. And the worst thing about it is that it makes you feel out of control.

I'll talk more about this in more detail later, but eating slowly puts you in the moment and takes you out of that zoned-out state — somewhere in between the waiter bringing you your plate and the wreckage you see when he comes back to get it.

Eating slowly puts you in control of the whole experience, lessens the perceived power you think food has over you, and helps you actually enjoy what you're eating.

4. Allow yourself to eat anything. If you decided to eat nothing but Snickers bars for a month, you not only wouldn't die, but depending on how many you ate, you could actually lose weight.

Trying "not to" eat certain foods makes those foods highly desirable. And the more you resist something, the more power it has over you.

But allowing yourself to eat all the foods you think you aren't supposed to eat takes the element of fear out of the equation. If you allow yourself to eat pasta, pasta is no longer scary. And when it stops being something you have to resist so strongly, it never becomes that thing you're desperate to have.

Allowing yourself to eat all the forbidden foods also allows you to figure out how you feel while you're eating them. It helps you eat more slowly since you're not looking at it as giving in to temptation and then bingeing on it like it's the last thing you'll ever eat.

When you allow yourself to eat ice cream sandwiches, you'll quickly figure out how gross they actually make you feel — a distinction you can't make when you're setting them up in a fearful way and then scarfing them down and calling yourself a pig afterward.

———————

The best approach to getting rid of resistance is not to create it in the first place. But if it's already there, you have to stop fighting the things that make you feel that way.

Be kind to yourself instead of critical of yourself. Appreciate the body you have instead of trying to force it into the one you want. Learn to enjoy eating instead of being scared of food and using it to make yourself feel better.

I promise you that if you do these exercises, you will have taken an enormous leap in progress toward your weight-loss goal. This is what I mean when I say that you can watch the weight lose itself.

It's insane that we never realize how much we're actually working against ourselves in our attempts at losing weight. These mental and physical shifts are critical and so much more powerful than doing things like cutting carbs and juicing all week.

Talking about resistance is the perfect segue to the next chapter: why diets don't work. That's because diets are all about resistance. And the sooner you stop buying them (and buying into them), the faster you can actually start moving forward and stop staying stuck right where you are.

Why Diets Don't Work

Losing weight is not the hard part.
The hard part is living with a diet for years.
— *Tommy Tomlinson*

I have tried every diet imaginable.

Actually, to be more accurate, I tried every diet that was ever created up until 2004, when I finally quit.

I started dieting when I was twelve years old. At the time, I didn't try an actual diet — I just stopped eating. The first real diet I ever went on was SlimFast. My mother had some in her cabinet and I started using it, probably when I was about thirteen.

From that point on, it was a free-for-all. I did the grapefruit diet, where all you eat is grapefruit and cottage cheese. I did NutriSystem with all the prepackaged meals. I did the cabbage soup diet. I did Richard Simmons's Deal-A-Meal. I took Dexatrim for about a year in the ninth grade back when it was basically meth. By the time I went off to college and still nothing was working, I started bingeing and purging.

I dieted, I binged, I purged, I starved myself, I over exercised. None of it ever worked.

And guess what? It never, ever occurred to me that it was because diets don't work. I thought it was me.

Because the diets all looked so different, it must be me, right? I mean, it was because I couldn't stick to one of them long enough to be successful. How could it not be me if every diet I ever went on ultimately ended because I lost control and binged?

Even though diets look different on the surface, deep down they're all the same. And the traits they all share are why they fail.

The reason diets look different is that diet makers have to keep changing them in order to sell them. And they all promise you that the one thing that makes them different is why they work. You've never seen anything like this! The revolutionary new system/ingredient/method — whatever.

And when the diet fails, you are the failure.

Yet you keep buying into the fantasy and thinking your dream will come true. It's like believing that there's a Prince Charming out there who will sweep you off your feet and that you'll live happily ever after — and that there will be no snoring, no fights over who left the cap off the toothpaste, or no laundry that you get stuck with and no one helps you with. That it'll all be okay once you get the ring. And when it doesn't work out, you blame yourself for not being good enough to make it work.

Living a healthy life — especially if you've trained yourself to engage in habits that are far from healthy — is messy, filled with hits and misses, and takes practice. All of this means that you will most definitely "fail" somewhere along the way. You don't live a perfectly healthy life 24-7, and you're not a failure if sometimes you do things that aren't in the least bit healthy.

Not only that, your body doesn't have to be sculpted into perfection for you to be acceptable. It enrages me how devastating an effect all the pictures of fashion models had on my fragile self-esteem growing up. This was way before we were all wise to the careful art of airbrushing. In my mind, Cindy Crawford was the most perfect creature on the planet. I used to stare at photos of her and think, "Why can't I look like that?" (Mercifully, I read somewhere recently that she has said, "I wish *I* looked like Cindy Crawford.")

Anyway, dieting is the equivalent of self-esteem destruction. It's the false fantasy you latch onto to magically transform yourself into a person in a magazine who doesn't even really look like that. And when you come up short, you're left with the same problem — only now you are even less confident than you were before because you failed. Which means you're even less likely to figure all this out. Which is why I'm writing this book.

Once again, weight is a symptom of the problem: emotional eating. And emotional eating is disordered eating.

Disordered eating and dieting go hand in hand. Eating in a disordered way ultimately stems from filling an internal void with food, which means you use food to shove down your pain instead of working through it. If you shove down pain long enough, your true voice can't speak.

Over time, all this adds up to a lack of self-worth and a belief that you're powerless to make changes. Dieting is the perfect go-to if you don't believe in your own power to solve a problem — you're exchanging your power for something you believe will solve your problem for you.

And worse, you're not even identifying what the real problem is. And in continuing to attack the weight, which means all you're focused on is what you look like, you erode your self-esteem even more.

Not only that, dieting reinforces the distorted relationship you already have with food. It trains you to see foods independently of each other rather than working together to nourish you. They are either good or bad, they should be included or avoided.

Dieting disconnects you from the experience of eating and makes food your adversary. And seeing food as something fearful fuels the binge eating/dieting cycle, which keeps you stuck in failure, which keeps you focused on the weight, which reinforces the distorted relationship you have with food and with your body.

Ultimately, dieting is like trying to use a Band-Aid to stop the flow of blood from a gaping wound. And when one Band-Aid doesn't work, you try another — and another and another. And when none of them work, you blame yourself for not applying them the right way — instead of wondering whether a Band-Aid is what you needed in the first place.

Now let's look at the exact reasons that diets don't work. Let's see what they all have in common that makes them (not you) the epic failures they all are.

Too much, too soon

Dieting requires you to make too many changes, all at once, in no time flat.

Real change involves learning, and to learn, you have to go through the process of trial and error. You have to take it one change at a time to figure out what works and what doesn't, what you're doing wrong, and how you can improve. Also, you have to understand why you're doing what you're doing in the first place and fix that — and you can't do this if you're distracted by trying to change everything you do.

Making a ton of changes all at the same time doesn't allow you the space to figure anything out. It would be like going to your first therapy appointment and walking out with a checklist that says quit drinking, make amends with your sister, change your friend group, and heal your inner child. And assuming that all those things don't have a thousand steps and feeling like you have to do all of them this week.

Making even one of those changes could take weeks or even years. And that's not a bad thing . . . that's actually the point. It's called a change, not a miracle. And change takes time.

To make a change that actually sticks, you have to first understand the mechanics of the behavior you're trying to change and why you have the behavior in the first place. Too often, we miss this critical step. We go from engagement to shame without figuring out where the behavior is coming from, how it developed, what steps are involved in it, what you're thinking about when you do it, and what triggers are pushing you to engage in it.

For example, binge eating. As I said earlier, you binge eat for a reason. You have to first see it for what it is. It's not you being a loser who has no control. I'm binge eating . . . why? Figure out the why. Then work on changing that. While you're doing that, figure out what the stressors are that lead you to the binge. Then work on changing those. And what do you binge on? Make some small changes to the foods you choose.

Most significantly, what do you think about while you're bingeing? How do you feel before, during, and after? There are goldmines of information in this step that you can use to help you change how you eat and ultimately stop binge eating.

Some of the modifications you try will work, some won't. Keep it up. After a while, you'll alter that behavior into something better — the behavior will change. Keep engaging in the new behavior and you'll eventually have a habit.

This process also holds true for the positive changes you want to make. If you want to eat more fruits and vegetables, it doesn't make sense to overload your fridge with everything from the produce section. You have to start slowly and eat more of the ones you currently like. Then you gradually add in new fruits and vegetables, figuring out which ones you enjoy and which ones you don't. Then you experiment with cooking with these new foods. If you try to do all of this at once, you'll give up and fail. (And you'll end up wasting a ton of money on produce that goes bad.)

A diet requires you to do things like throw all the carbs out of your house when all you currently eat is bread and pasta. Then you're supposed to adhere to an extensive, detailed menu of the specific foods you must eat for the next two weeks, even though you've never eaten half of them. And the menu consists of foods your husband and your kids may hate or not be in the mood for every single night — oh yeah, and you also hardly ever cook. Finally, don't forget to use one scoop of this enzyme-loaded powder with green tea extract in your fruit smoothie every morning or none of it will work.

Is it any wonder we never stick to a diet? Who could do all these things at once? And even if you were able to, what happens when it's over? You go right back to doing what you were before the diet. You have the exact same habits you've always had — and when you do what you've always done, you get what you've always gotten.

Unless you plan on staying locked in your house for the rest of time, you won't be able to sustain diets that force you into making multiple, radical changes — because they don't work in the real world. The only people diets do work for are celebrities who have personal chefs who make all their meals, each with the perfect nutrient profile to ensure zero cellulite, shiny hair, clear skin, and an amazing sex life. These people can make tons of changes all at once because they don't have to make choices — they have other people do it for them. So, stop being brainwashed to believe that you're a loser because you don't do what Kim K does. Because Kim K has a team of people following her around, telling her what to do.

Changing everything you do all at once is unsustainable, particularly when the changes involve doing the complete opposite of the habits you've taken a lifetime to establish. Trying to change multiple behaviors at once is overwhelming and takes away the feeling of control you need to persevere and make lasting changes.

Furthermore, a change that becomes a habit is one in which distinctions were made during the process of making the change. That's the trial-and-error part I mentioned. Distinctions are made over time — not in the next two weeks.

So, making too many changes, all at once, leads to nothing but overwhelm, stress, and giving up. In other words, failure.

All-or-nothing

Hand-in-hand with the too much, too soon trait of dieting is the all-or-nothing mentality you must adopt while you're on one.

The all-or-nothing approach is near and dear to my heart, because I have a huge tendency to go all in whenever I do anything. And although it seems like a good thing on the surface, it usually sets you up for failure.

This is especially true with dieting, because when you're not able to sustain this level of action-taking, you end up feeling like a failure and tell yourself how weak you are for not being able to stick with it.

If I decide that I'm going to go all in on making sure I get my kids safely to school while I'm driving, that's a good thing. It's easy to do the right things in this scenario because they don't involve willpower (more on that in a minute), and missing one of the steps doesn't mean I don't have what it takes to be successful at this goal — it just means I forgot. I make them put on their seatbelts, I make sure my littlest one rides in the back seat and not the front, I drive the speed limit, and I don't run red lights. And if I miss a step — if I go too fast on a morning when we're late — I don't say forget it and become totally reckless from then on out.

If you say you're not going to eat carbs for a week, when you slip up and eat a Hershey's Kiss, you tend to go all-or-nothing in the opposite direction: you throw in the towel and finish the entire bag. If you say you're going to run every day this week, when you miss a day, you stop working out altogether. When you say you're not going to snack between lunch and dinner and you mindlessly grab one of your kid's potato chips, you binge eat for the rest of the day.

For any goal that is related to self-improvement, all-or-nothing is a dangerous approach to take. Working on yourself means your self-esteem is involved — which means your inner critic is on the sidelines waiting for you to fail. And all-or-nothing requires perfection, so anything short of that equals failure. Then your inner critic starts talking, and if you're not paying attention, you'll be absorbing her every word. Then you give up completely and go all-or-nothing in the opposite direction.

The truth is, improving yourself can be accomplished in a multitude of ways, all of which may consist of numerous tiny steps. And some of those steps may or may not work for you and your lifestyle. So just because it worked for someone else doesn't mean it will work for you. And just because it doesn't, that doesn't mean you failed.

The all-or-nothing dieting approach to losing weight sets you up for a pressure-filled, miserable experience that ultimately results in failure and puts you back at square one (minus another shred of self-confidence). If you want to permanently lose weight you have to be willing to sacrifice the immediate gratification mindset. You have to be willing to switch your approach from all-or-nothing to patiently and consistently making small, consistent changes over time.

Gaining small wins from successfully making them builds your confidence, which is what you need to continue and reinforce the certainty that you can do this all on your own, without relying on a diet to do it for you.

The need for willpower

In our culture, we celebrate success. And success means doing whatever it takes to get results.

So, we celebrate people who push themselves, who constantly strive to achieve, who work hard to beat their competitors. We celebrate people who work around the clock, who don't sleep, who force themselves to keep going. We celebrate people who seem to have a never-ending supply of willpower and who consistently use it.

In fact, all of us — not just the ultra-successful — have become so accustomed to using willpower to get things done that we hardly even notice we're doing it. It's just a way of life.

But the problem with approaching life this way is that we tend to put people in one of two groups: the ones who have what it takes and the others who don't. But willpower isn't a personality trait. The truth is that anyone can use willpower — and all of us do at some point.

Remember Sir Isaac Newton's third law of physics: for every action, there is an equal and opposite reaction. So, using willpower ultimately results in a counterbalance of backing off. Using willpower takes energy, and in this case the energy is forcing yourself to do something you don't want to do or don't feel like doing. So, when the resistance becomes too great, you must neutralize it.

At its foundation, dieting is all about willpower. You're forcing yourself to do things — a lot of them — that you don't usually do. Loading yourself up with ten changes that you have to make to be successful at the diet requires an almost Herculean amount of effort. So, coming up with this much willpower is not just challenging, it's utterly overwhelming.

Diets don't mention any of this, of course. But the unspoken truth about all of them is this: if you can come up with enough willpower, you'll succeed. And if you can't, you'll fail. You just didn't have what it takes.

But the thing about willpower is that is that it eventually runs out. You can't sustain it forever. It isn't an unlimited resource, and it eventually runs out. And there is research to back this up.

The academic term for a decrease in willpower over time is *ego depletion*. Although there is conflicting evidence for the concept that using willpower over time decreases your capacity to exercise it, most of the research indicates that willpower is a limited resource.

In a study conducted by Roy Baumeister[1], a social psychologist, during his tenure at Case Western Reserve University, participants were placed in a room and given a puzzle to solve. Before working on it, half of the participants were presented with a bowl of radishes and a plate of freshly baked chocolate chip cookies. They were asked to refrain from eating the cookies and forced to eat the radishes instead. The other half of the participants were allowed to eat the cookies.

The participants who had to eat the radishes and resist the cookies spent less time trying to solve the puzzle and made fewer attempts at solving it than those who were allowed to eat the cookies. The conclusion drawn was that the participants forced to abstain from eating the cookies were mentally fatigued from exercising willpower and had less capacity to stick with the puzzle.

Although this theory has been tested to determine its validity and the results are mixed, I think it's worth considering. After all, I don't need a laboratory experiment to validate the fact that I'm much more capable of using willpower to eat better earlier in the day than I am after a hectic day of working, mothering, and housekeeping.

---

[1] Baumeister RF, Bratslavsky E, Muraven M, Tice DM. Ego depletion: is the active self a limited resource? J Pers Soc Psychol 1998;74(5):1252-65.

Whether you're a unicorn who's adept at using willpower at all hours of the day or whether you seem to run out of it as the day goes on, there's no point in calling yourself a loser when you don't have enough of it.

The truth is that dieting requires you to spend a huge amount of time and energy thinking about food and what you're allowed to eat and how much of it you can eat, and this is mentally exhausting. Not only that, if you've trained yourself to eat when you're feeling any kind of resistance, the combination of mental fatigue and the stress you feel during a typical day usually leads to bingeing.

However, if you've set your environment up properly (meaning you make it easy, not hard, for you to make healthy choices) and you aren't forcing yourself into a battle with food, there's no need for willpower and you're more likely to be successful.

Using willpower also conditions you to think of food in terms of being "good" or "bad," and this way of thinking is what keeps you in an adversarial relationship with food, which in turn fuels your disordered eating.

To use a real-world example, think about what we do during the holidays. During the holidays, we eat as if it's our last meal. And it's because of using so much willpower and working so hard at being "good" during the regular days that we go all out during holiday celebrations. We load up huge plates of food, scarf them down, and feel like crap afterward. And we actually look forward to holidays precisely for that reason.

Even though it feels miserable to be stuffed and bloated, we're so relieved to not have to be so rigid. We're relieved to not have to use willpower. So, we dive headfirst into a downward slide of bingeing — which we'll then try to make up for with a massive show of willpower once the holidays have ended. But maybe if we didn't have to use so much willpower the rest of the year, eating in a normal way wouldn't be so challenging during the holidays.

And back to the point of seeing foods as "good" or "bad." The foods we choose to fill our plates up with during any holiday are the ones we're not supposed to eat. Mashed potatoes loaded with butter and cheese at Thanksgiving, bags of miniature chocolates during Halloween, huge plates of barbecue on the Fourth of July, seconds of pie or cake at Christmas.

However, if we chose to see these foods differently, it wouldn't be like this. If we saw them not as these massively tempting foods that we had to force ourselves to stay away from and never eat, if we actually allowed ourselves to eat them every once in a while during the year, we'd see them as occasionally enjoyable and not all that "comforting." Actually, we'd figure out pretty quickly that they don't really make us feel that great — especially when we binge on them.

(Side note: since my binges used to consist of anything chocolate, Halloween was a free-for-all for me. Once I realized that I could always go to the store on November 1st and buy bags of miniature candy bars if I felt like it, I stopped viewing the holiday as some sort of opportunity to overdose on chocolate that only came around once a year.)

Using willpower long-term doesn't work. Therefore, dieting doesn't either.

Trying "not to"

Trying "not to" is a huge part of why diets don't work.

You've probably heard the phrase, "What you think about, you bring about." I believe this to be absolutely true. And although I'm not a physicist, I've seen enough proof of this concept in my own life to validate it.

Trying not to do something keeps your attention focused on whatever it is you're trying not to do. If you're trying not to eat carbs, all you'll think about all day are the carbs you're not supposed to eat.

The entire time you diet, you keep yourself in a state of trying "not to" — of avoiding, resisting, abstaining from, and eliminating. Even if the diet tells you that you can do something, it's phrased as "you're allowed to." And making certain foods acceptable means that others are not.

The tricky part is that one diet will include only these foods, while another diet will tell you that those same foods are terrible for you — sometimes to the point that you become afraid of them. And then all you see on the news for a whole year is how nightshade vegetables will corrode your insides and why you should avoid them like the plague — especially because that's what Tom and Giselle do.

This whole negative-focused approach that goes with dieting also exaggerates your language and heightens the fear we associate with food. We rarely see things for what they are, because we've created a huge drama around eating.

So, you see a plate of fries and proclaim, "I can just look at those and gain weight" or feel like you have to summon all your strength to resist them. Instead of calmly assessing the situation, knowing that every time you scarf down a bunch of fries you feel physically heavy afterward and then choosing not to eat them — or to eat them, if that's what you really want to do — you engage in a mental battle and can't focus on anything until you give into the urge . . . and then binge eat the whole plate.

But when you start seeing all foods as acceptable to eat rather than off-limits or "bad," an interesting thing happens. Rather than having it turn into a free-for-all, it's the opposite. When you allow yourself to eat anything you want, you'll actually eat less. That's because there won't be any resistance to overcome. And by eliminating fear from the equation, you'll be more in control and won't have the urge to binge as often.

Then the feeling of control you have helps you assess what's happening and see it more clearly. Instead of feeling the urge to binge and immediately reacting to it, you can say, "Ok, I feel like bingeing on these potato chips, but I know what this feeling is and exactly what's going to happen if I give in to it. I'm going to feel miserable afterward, and it's just not worth it."

Then you don't go around all day reacting to every feeling you have and intensifying the fear-based relationship you've developed with food. You put yourself in control.

In contrast, the can't/don't negative-focused dieting mentality takes you out of the driver's seat and makes food in control of you.

One size fits all

This is one of the worst aspects of diets: they're one-size-fits-all. However, for some reason, we all look past it.

All these different women — who have different day-to-day lives, who are in different phases of their lives, and who have different preferences and tastes — all go on the same diet and expect to get the same results.

It's crazy, right?

You don't wear the same style of clothes your best friend does — and if you do, you probably don't wear the same brand, shop at the same store, or wear the same accessories. That's because you have a different body type, you like neutrals instead of bright colors, and you have more or less money to spend. Maybe you don't even know that much about fashion — maybe it's a lot easier for your friend to put things together than it is for you. Can you imagine a stylist giving you the same wardrobe as your friend and expecting to be satisfied with the way you look?

Or imagine a doctor who gives all of his patients the same prescription without giving anyone a physical or assessing their medical history. And then telling the people who don't get better that the reason they're still sick is that they didn't take their pills.

You would never go back to a doctor who practiced that way, yet we all keep dieting because we're all willing to gloss over this obvious flaw in exchange for the fantasy that this is the one diet that will finally work.

So even if a diet worked for your next-door neighbor (and don't forget, even if it did, she's going to put the weight back on if she didn't change any of her habits), maybe that's because she has a housekeeper and therefore has time for an hour-long workout every day. Maybe her two children are in high school and don't need the hands-on care that your two toddlers do. Maybe her husband loves to cook, and he's delighted to help prepare the special meals required on the diet. Or maybe he's delighted to help with the kids while she does.

Despite this, you're watching the video of the people who got these amazing results, and you're promised the same ones if you just go on this diet. And when you don't get the same results, it's because you weren't as diligent or consistent as they were. You didn't work hard enough.

What's more likely is that you worked plenty hard enough — but maybe your schedule made it difficult to prepare every single dish that was required, or maybe you have a family to feed and they don't like salmon or green juice, or maybe you don't live near a boutique grocery store that sells flax oil. A diet factors none of these things in.

But aside from the differences in daily schedules, life phases, and individual preferences, the biggest issue with the one-size-fits-all approach to dieting is that it never addresses the habits you have.

Diets aren't about modifying behaviors — they're about following instructions. So, none of your habits ever change as part of a diet. And habits are as individual as outfits. Your habits vary radically from those of your friends. Even if you're a binge eater, you probably binge on different foods and your triggers are different. What has to change are the behaviors, the thoughts that go with them,

63

and the environmental and emotional triggers that push you to engage in them.

One-size-fits-all doesn't work for anything in life if you really think about it. It's why this term is usually used in a derogatory fashion. But the most damaging aspect of this approach is that because we choose to remain oblivious to it, we blame ourselves when it doesn't work for us — instead of recognizing the absurdity of expecting it to work in the first place.

Disconnection

Many of the characteristics of dieting that we've just covered result in you being disconnected from the food you eat and the experience of eating itself. This in turn reinforces the adversarial relationship you've already developed with food and the fear you associate with eating.

When you have an adversarial relationship with food, you're more likely to binge eat. That's because when you categorize foods as "good" or "bad," the implication is that you don't have enough control to choose for yourself. And when you label foods as "bad," you're increasing the likelihood that you will eat those very foods when you can no longer withstand the resistance you've built toward them.

So, your already adversarial relationship with food — which is established by viewing foods as having power over you and then having to use willpower not to eat them — is reinforced by dieting, because this is exactly what dieting consists of. So, the more you diet, the more you fuel your disconnected relationship with food.

A major issue with this is that having this kind of relationship with food starts to look normal. And the dieting industry capitalizes on this fear we have of food. It sets up entire categories of food as off-limits and in extreme cases actually prepares the meals for you, taking you and your ability to choose completely out of the equation.

Here's an example from my own life. When I was in college, I signed up for Nutrisystem. If you don't remember, it's a program that delivered low-calorie prepackaged meals you ate for a few weeks to lose weight. Each meal came in a microwaveable plastic container that was about the size of an iPad. No preparation was involved — you just heated it up, ripped off the cellophane, and ate.

There was no enjoyment in eating these meals. I was completely and totally disconnected from the food I was eating. The elements of preference, choice, and preparation were eliminated from this interaction between me and the "food." I would hardly even call it food. I didn't choose what to prepare, I didn't go to the store and read a label or pick ingredients that were the freshest, I didn't handle the foods while cooking them, and I didn't sit down and enjoy the meal I prepared for myself. There was zero enjoyment.

The food was actually an afterthought. My only motivation for doing the program was to prevent myself from overeating. Unfortunately, this doesn't work very well when you can't stop yourself from eating three meals at once. I ate one, then another, and then another until I felt full. Needless to say, NutriSystem was yet another diet that I failed to stick to.

This entire experience was based in fear — fear of losing control. But that's exactly what I did. I lost control because I knew I was supposed to eat only one, but the "experience" of eating that one meal was so utterly unsatisfying, I needed another one.

The reason I signed up for that program was obviously to lose weight. But the weight was there because I ate in a disordered way — I had taught myself to binge to fill the inner void I had. But since I had never addressed the real problem, I was continuing to binge eat. And this program that I bought into to keep myself from overeating didn't work, because my urge to binge wasn't satisfied.

And of course, I shamed myself relentlessly for not even being able to be successful on a program that couldn't have dumbed it down more to keep me from eating too much.

I can't think of a better way to disconnect someone from the experience of eating than to take real food, freeze dry it, put it in a plastic container covered with cellophane, and have them heat it up in a microwave. And then sell it solely based on the number of calories it has in an effort to get you to eat less.

Even when diet makers don't sell actual food, their message of food being something you have no control over and that you have to avoid disconnects you from it. Food is something that nourishes you — not something that works against you or that you should fear. And if the food isn't particularly nourishing, then it's probably something you shouldn't eat very often.

When you lessen the power you've given food over you, you'll no longer be afraid of losing control when you encounter it or be terrified of eating the wrong things. Then you'll begin to see eating as a pleasurable experience and will then be more likely to cook more and experiment with new foods and try new things. At that point, food will no longer be your adversary.

When you get to enjoy what you're eating, you're relaxed and engaged with the whole process: preparing your food, cooking it, sharing it, eating it. When you make eating an experience, you tend to eat more slowly because you appreciate the effort you put into making the meal and want to enjoy it more. And if you eat slowly, you're more aware of feeling full — and then you can stop when you are.

This is in sharp contrast to feeling out of control around food and then inhaling it when you're presented with it.

Food is part of nature, and so are we. To get a little deep, you and the food you eat are part of the same energy. When you set up a fear-based relationship with food and you try not to eat it — which is

66

exactly what you do when you diet — you are essentially disconnecting with yourself. And if you disconnect with yourself, you will never be able to change the body you live in.

Being aware of how dieting creates such a powerful disconnection between you and food is critically important. If you don't ever see this, you will remain forever stuck in the dieting loop.

Tell me what to do

When I first became a dietitian, I had people constantly ask me to come up with meal plans for them.

I couldn't put my finger on it, but I didn't like doing it because I somehow knew that it wasn't going to work. So even though I reluctantly gave them what they asked for, my heart wasn't in it.

After doing this for several years, I finally figured out why passing out random three-day menus never works long-term. That's because following instructions never helps people make real changes.

If I tell you exactly what to eat for the next week, you may be able to do it. But after the week is over, have you changed anything about what you usually do? Have you learned how to eat differently? Have you learned anything?

The answer is a resounding no.

And, once again, if I have three days' worth of menus that provide the perfect balance of nutrients, is that meal plan going to work for your sister who lives a totally different life than you do? Even if I tailored it for each of you to meet each of your energy requirements based on your current weight, the same menu isn't going to be as easy to follow for you if your life is way more hectic than your sister's. And it won't work at all for your sister if she's lactose intolerant and most of the recipes contain cheese.

Preferences and ease of implementation aside, neither of you will have changed anything about the way you eat after the three days are over. And then you're both back to square one.

Furthermore, me telling you what to do absolves you of any responsibility for figuring out what's healthy, how to incorporate it into your daily life, and how to make those changes stick. All of which require a period of trial and error that's required for learning.

Remember, it's not about what you eat — it's about the way that you eat it. The what comes later. So even if I gave you a year of menus and you followed them to the letter (doubtful), you still wouldn't have changed how you eat. And you'll go right back to doing what you've always done: eat to fill an emotional void. You'll still use food as a reward, to make yourself feel better, to neutralize pain.

So, when you go on a diet, you put yourself in the vulnerable position of having someone tell you what to do instead of making your own changes. It's a vulnerable position because in effect you're saying you can't do it yourself, which isn't true at all. You're putting yourself in a place of desperation, which means you've given away all your power.

It may not feel like it, but you have the power to not only make changes, but to also live a completely different life than you're living. You would shock yourself at the things you're capable of. Spending your life on a diet trying to lose weight is living in such a small way that it's tragic.

You have power to change the way you eat, to change your habits, to change your life. But you can't do any of these things as long as you're relying on me or a diet to tell you what to do.

You have to take responsibility for making your own changes. And that's a real step into vulnerability, because once you take responsibility, there's no one to blame.

The irony in all this, of course, is when you fail at another diet, you blame yourself anyway. But when you put yourself in a position of power over your own life and you "fail," you're far less likely to take such a hit to your confidence, because you built it up just by taking charge in the first place.

The amazing thing about taking responsibility for making your own changes is that you don't see it as failure when you slip up and one of your changes doesn't work. You'll start to see it as part of the learning and growing process.

You'll also see that there are an infinite number of changes you can make. So, if one change isn't working — if it's too challenging at this point or if it doesn't fit with your life and your individual preferences — you move on to another one. Or keep making slight modifications to it until you've mastered it.

Once you master a change and repeat it, you create a habit. And when you create a series of habits, you create a new life.

If I give you a meal plan, none of this happens. And a diet is nothing more than one big meal plan — only it comes with the false promise that it will change your life. So, let's talk about that.

The Magic Pill

And now we've come to the most destructive aspect of dieting. And it's also the biggest reason why they don't ever work.

What's behind every diet is the belief that there is some sort of magic solution that will fix everything for you. Diet makers all promise you that theirs is the only one that really works, and this implies that there is only one solution — you just haven't found it yet. Even worse, they not only promise you weight loss, they promise you that a better, more beautiful life will be yours once you lose the weight.

Neither of these things — the magic solution or the perfect life it promises — exist.

Losing weight won't bring you anything other than a body that weighs less, and the more you buy into the concept that shedding the weight will somehow magically change your life, the longer you will stay stuck searching for another diet that promises the same thing, just in a different-looking package.

As you've just learned in this chapter, diets will never, ever work. And they don't for all the reasons I've just given. Ultimately, they all have the same basic structure, and it's flawed.

But not only do none of them work, they render you powerless. That's because as soon as you start a new diet, what you're essentially doing is telling yourself that you can't do it. You're subconsciously giving away your power.

Making yourself powerless destroys your self-confidence. And you must have confidence in yourself if you're going to make real changes in your life. You have to have confidence to keep going when you stumble or make a mistake. Again, making changes that last is a messy process that requires you to accept your mistakes and see them as opportunities to learn — to figure out what works for you and what doesn't.

You have to have confidence to see this process in a whole new way: to see it as a journey and not an overnight success. To see it as making an investment in yourself rather than winning the lottery.

And you also have to have confidence in yourself if you're going to love yourself for where you are right now, in the body you're currently in. And the only way to do that is to understand that you're in this place because of everything you've experienced up to this point — good and bad. And that cannot *not* be beautiful.

All of this is shattered when you tell yourself that you can't live your life until you've lost weight. That you hate the way you look and need to drop the weight as soon as possible to look beautiful. That losing weight will make you more worthy. And that if you could just finally lose it, everything about your life would change.

This is the soul-destroying fantasy you're buying into every time you start a new diet. The fantasy they're selling you isn't real, and whatever way they promise to bring the fantasy to life is destined to fail.

This is at the heart of what makes dieting so destructive. You're giving your power over to something that won't ultimately work, so when it's over you're not only powerless — you're a failure, too. And then you're even more susceptible to the illusion and more desperate to make it a reality the next time around.

Your belief in the fantasy fuels your desperation — and that's exactly how diet makers want you to feel. Because the more desperate you are, the more likely you are to buy what they're selling. That's why they promote their products so relentlessly via this illusion of a better life.

Another big problem with the magic pill scenario is that it absolves you from taking responsibility for yourself and doing the hard work necessary to make real changes. When you go on a diet, you're relying on someone to tell you what to do. You want someone to give you the set of instructions to follow instead of learning how to eat differently. You're asking someone to wave a magic wand and make ten, twenty, or even thirty years of bad habits disappear for a few weeks, so you can get rid of the evidence of those habits — only to have them return full force once the diet's over.

You can't start the process of real change until you accept where you are, why you are here, and that you got yourself here. Once you accept that it's up to you, that's when you get your power back. And when you take responsibility, there can be no more excuses. It feels scary to let go of all your excuses, but the power you claim by taking responsibility is enough to wipe out your need to keep hiding behind them.

The weight is there because of your unique drivers that make you eat the way you do. You have to change the thoughts that make you eat this way, because those are what lead to the habits that create the excess weight. You have to learn how to take control of your environment to manage the triggers that cause you to binge eat. You have to be willing to go through the process of trial and error that results in massive changes in your thoughts and habits and learn from the insights you gain during the process.

And during this process, you will start to see yourself differently and ultimately become who you were meant to be. This, not weight loss, is what changes your life.

You can't diet your way to a better life — but you can get the life you want by using what you already have inside of you to create it.

———————

Dieting isn't ever going to work, it's pointless and completely destructive to keep doing it, it will keep you imprisoned and stuck in failure, and it will continue to wreck your self-esteem. And the longer you keep doing it, the more you'll keep searching for that one special version that will finally work — and you'll wake up one morning when you're 60, wondering where your life went.

The sooner you accept that no diet is ever going to work, the sooner you can start your hike down the long, winding path toward health. This path isn't always easy to see, and you'll veer off it every once in a while. But if you train yourself to get back on it, eventually you'll see results.

The thing about this path is that you have to make a commitment to take it. It's not the smooth, easy-to-follow track lane that leads directly to a finish line in record time. (A finish line that you'll never cross.) No one is going to help you to the end, because no one can — everyone's path is different.

There are tools you can use to make your way down the path, and those are what I'm going to give you. But the reality is that there's no one path to travel — and there's also no final destination.

I'm hoping at this point that you're ready to give up on dieting take responsibility for your life. But before we continue, I want to tell you my story and how I figured all this out.

Trust me, I learned the hard way. And I want to tell you the whole painful story, so you don't have to spend 25 years of your life trying to figure it out like I did. I also want to inspire you, so that you know you're not alone and that someone out there truly understands how you feel.

My Story

Even though I am a registered dietitian, my academic credentials are not what makes me an expert on losing weight. What makes me truly an expert is that I spent more than two decades of my life, trying everything imaginable to lose weight — until I finally figured out that everything I was doing was wrong.

I already mentioned a little bit about how I grew up and how my relationship with food developed. I received mixed messages when it came to food from an early age. We all absorb the environment around us, and growing up in the late 70s/early 80s created a highly distorted relationship with food and with my body that would haunt me for years to come.

Little girls' behaviors are without a doubt deeply influenced by those of their mothers. And I don't know one mom of that generation that didn't talk about being fat and who didn't diet.

The diets back then had little to no nutritional basis, nor did they support a healthy relationship with food or eating. Basically, the message was to eat as little as possible to lose as much weight as possible. So, my mom did what all women during that time did: she drank a ton of Tab, ate diet bars and drank diet shakes, and barely ate anything resembling real food. The goal was to be skinny and do it as fast as possible.

But before I became aware that I should eat less to make myself look better, I had taught myself how to eat to make myself feel better.

Before my teenage years, when the knowledge hit me that I shouldn't eat too much, food was always available, and I ate as much of it as I wanted. As I got older, however, I quickly became aware that eating too much was unacceptable.

During my teenage years, I knew that food was something to be scared of and that I should feel shame at eating more than I should. But I had a few vivid food-related experiences early on that primed me for that experience.

I vividly remember being out to eat at a restaurant with my parents and some of their friends. I suppose I was in the sixth or seventh grade — not a teenager yet, but self-conscious enough to feel embarrassed at being paid attention to, especially in a negative way. I was used to loading my plate up at home at any hour of the day with whatever I wanted. So, when the breadbasket came my way that night, I held on to it.

The adults were talking and didn't notice for a while. But after I had eaten three or four pieces of bread, my father scolded me from across the table to "leave some for everyone else." I can still feel the tremendous shame I experienced. (He, of course, wasn't intending to shame me, but I felt ashamed nonetheless.)

It was obvious to me from that experience that eating too much was not only socially unacceptable but, worse, a reflection of what kind of person you are. In that moment, a belief took shape deep within me that eating too much made you unacceptable to others and that overeating, especially in public, was something to be embarrassed about. So, I realized that if I was going to eat to make myself feel better, I had better stay out of sight.

The older I got, the messages I got from adults about food and eating became more negative. Whereas food was always available to me as a child, it was now talked about as something I should be careful about, if not downright afraid of. People started warning me that certain foods were "fattening" and that they would do things like "stick to my hips."

My mother still allowed my brother and me to eat what we wanted, but now those foods came with admonitions not to eat too much of them. It was confusing, to say the least. Up until my early teenage years, no food was off limits. We were used to eating all kinds of bread, pasta with cheese, and any kind of packaged food you could think of. Then, all of a sudden, everything came with a warning.

I experienced this not only at home, but also among my friends. Not one of us was even close to being overweight, but you would never have guessed that by listening to us. It seemed as though overnight everyone had become acutely aware of this new universe in which we were all going to wake up fat. And I mean, there couldn't be anything worse than that.

Starting in about the ninth grade, we all got rid of the lunches our mothers had packed for us and bought a Diet Coke to drink instead. We took diet pills with our diet drinks and tried to make it through the afternoon. We endlessly picked apart our bodies, showing each other how "fat" we were, pinching ourselves in various places to emphasize how revolting we were.

However, with the exception of my mother's sporadic comments about some foods being fattening, nothing really changed with my eating habits at home. I starved myself all day at school then started bingeing as soon as I got off the bus. My brother and I had developed such a habit of eating anything we wanted all afternoon after school and into the evening that it was difficult to stop. But in my mind, I was balancing everything out during the day by not eating.

There is no doubt that I used food as a way to cope with the typical teenage challenges I experienced. I had no way of making sense of all the feelings of inadequacy I had; I didn't talk about them to anyone, so instead I just filled myself up with food. I shoved all my feelings and emotions down by eating. At the same time, I also was highly focused on getting my father's attention and approval, which was a tough thing to accomplish. Not because he didn't love me, but because he was so unbelievably busy. But even if I was able to somehow miraculously capture his attention, I was sure I wouldn't measure up.

My father's job required lots of entertaining, so there was always some sort of party or gathering at our house. And from overhearing hundreds of conversations among the guests, I came to understand that women who looked good were the most admired. Women in our Southern culture were not expected to do much, but the one thing they could get noticed for was by being attractive and, most of all, thin. So, I was determined to be one of those women. (More accurately, I was even more determined not to be the other type.)

The one thing that saved me during my teenage years was the fact that I was very active. Although I watched a ton of television, I also was involved in lots of activities outside of school. I was a cheerleader throughout high school and also began taking aerobics classes after school, which were the new thing in the mid-80s. I swam on the local swim team during most summers, and I ran cross country during my senior year. All this activity helped me balance out my radical eating behaviors.

However, the extreme disconnect I experienced between using food to self-medicate and the constant awareness that eating too much would make me physically unacceptable (and in my mind worthless) was damaging to my self-esteem. I wasn't consciously aware of this internal struggle, and it manifested as a persistent, nagging question that took years to eliminate: *What is wrong with me?*

When I went to college, everything fell apart. Even though my eating habits were out of control as I was growing up, at least there was some sort of routine to my days. When I went away that first year, I had no structure, nothing to rein in my compulsive behaviors. Everything was new — the schedule, the people, the surroundings — and I was completely overwhelmed.

There is the old adage that girls go to college and gain the Freshman 15, which is fairly accurate. However, this dismissive phrase makes it sounds as if a few pounds is something harmless that has no effect on anything other than a scale. It doesn't come close to describing the feelings of self-hatred that came along with the extra weight that I gained that first year away from home.

I was a good student, but all of my self-worth was wrapped up in the way that I looked, so the extra weight to me meant that I was a failure. I can still remember sitting in my dorm room, barely even being able to look in the mirror I was so revolted by the way I looked. The feeling of shame was so overwhelming that the only thing I wanted to do was hide in my room and eat. And that's exactly what I did. I would go through the drive-through of a local fast-food restaurant and order enough food for three people. And I would return to my room, alone, and eat everything, which of course made me feel disgusting and more worthless.

Food was the only way I knew how to comfort myself, so when I felt the feelings of shame and failure as a result of gaining weight, I ate. Food was the only thing I had. When I tried to do better by not eating all the "wrong" foods or simply by not eating at all, the extreme discomfort I felt at depriving myself ultimately was too much to take, and I binged. Then I gained more weight and felt more shame and failure.

I tried diet after diet after diet, and of course nothing worked. I would diet some weight off, then when the diet was over, I went back to my old habits and I gained it all back. I alternated between relentlessly dieting and bingeing. I over exercised, and I continued taking diet pills. But nothing worked.

Then, a good friend of mine let me in on a little secret of hers. She told me that after she ate too much, it was super easy to fix. You just made yourself throw up. Once I figured out how to do this, I was liberated. I could keep my bingeing habit and not gain any weight. It was like a miracle. It was like being able to drink yourself into oblivion without ever having a hangover. She and I would hit every drive-through in town, loading up on as much food as we could get, eat all of it, and purge.

It was great to have someone who understood my compulsive need to eat and also my extreme desire to rid myself of the weight and be thin. However, the shame of being overweight was nothing compared to the feelings of absolute worthlessness I experienced after bingeing and purging.

I knew somehow in my heart that throwing up what I ate was about the most self-destructive thing I could do, both physically and psychologically. But the praise I received as a result of losing weight from friends and family was enough to keep my approval-seeking self stuck in this vicious cycle for years to come. So, I spent three years of college in this hideous downward spiral, continuing to binge and purge.

Looking back, it's easy to see how my earlier conditioning played right into my becoming bulimic. Eating alone to me was preferable to eating with others, which is particularly important if you are bingeing on food to fill an emotional void. I was used to eating alone and to hiding what I ate, so the isolation and secrecy required for being bulimic wasn't unusual to me.

Also, the feeling that eating is shameful and that your body itself is something to be ashamed of is a hallmark of bulimia — in fact, I believe it is the motivating force behind it. After all, there isn't a more extreme way to rid yourself of the food you just ate than by violently regurgitating it, and I think going to those lengths is an indicator of how someone feels, both about herself and about food.

Around the time I graduated from college and moved to Atlanta for my first job, I had decided that I was no longer capable of sustaining the abuse I was inflicting on myself. I had moved into an apartment by myself, so even though it would have been the perfect set-up for continuing with this destructive behavior, I decided to stop and find some other way to be thin. So, I returned to my other extreme behaviors.

I would drink diet soda all day, eating nothing, and have a Lean Cuisine for dinner. I hardly ever had lunch with my coworkers; I ran errands instead and attempted to focus on my work without eating anything at all. Once I got home, with nothing to sustain myself all day, I tried to do an exercise tape in my apartment before dinner. I could hardly make it half-way through without collapsing from exhaustion. Then, once I started on my 300-calorie, prepackaged dinner, I was unable to stop myself from eating two or three of them.

I can honestly say that the worst part about all of this misery had nothing to do with the extra weight. Nor did it have anything to do with the physical toll of all the abuse. Without question, the most devastating thing about my years of gaining weight, losing weight, and gaining it all back was the sense of worthlessness I carried with me.

I remember the day that something inside me changed. I was sitting in my tiny apartment on the couch, sobbing. I literally could not take the shame and the torture I had been enduring for one more minute. I knew that something had to change. I thought about all the extreme things I had done to just lose weight, once and for all, and how none of those things had worked. And I had always believed that the problem was me.

But now I started to think about how maybe the problem wasn't me — maybe it was my approach. Maybe I needed to just take a step back and take a breath. Maybe I needed to stop being so extreme. Maybe I needed to be nicer to myself. As I sat there and cried, I started to feel something shift. I felt lighter almost immediately. It didn't happen overnight, but letting go of all that mental weight was the catalyst that eventually helped me shed the physical weight.

I made a decision that day. It was a resolution to just start where I was and little by little begin to do the things that I knew were healthy — even if they didn't necessarily result in weight loss.

If it felt healthy to me mentally, I did it. If it felt good physically, I did it. If I felt like taking a walk around the block and get some fresh air, I did. If I felt like taking a nap, I did. If I felt like reading a book, I did. If I felt like doing nothing and staring out the window for a while, I did.

Basically, I just started being nice to myself. And treating myself in this new way started to slowly displace the feelings of striving, discomfort, anxiety, and misery that had been my standard for so many years.

I decided that I was going to stop trying to lose weight altogether. For someone who had built her whole life around the way that she looked and who had spent all of her mental, emotional, and physical energy trying to beat her body into submission, this was not an easy thing, to put it mildly.

However, I had reached my absolute limit of having tortured myself for so long that I really had no other choice. I decided that the pain of being overweight wasn't worth the pain I'd been inflicting on myself to not be that way. I decided that I'd rather be happy and joyful and weigh more than I wanted to than be miserable and suffer just so I could be ten pounds lighter.

I decided that I was going to treat myself the way I would want someone else to treat me. That instead of being my harshest critic, I would be my biggest supporter. That instead of setting for nothing less than perfection, I would just accept myself as good enough the way I was — and then work slowly and simply toward improving. I decided that maybe it wasn't all about being thin — maybe it was about being healthy.

I gave some serious thought to how I thought about food and my relationship to it. I realized that it was a fear-based, all-or-nothing relationship in which I had set up food as both the enemy and the ultimate friend. I realized that it was a relationship that was exaggerated in importance and founded on massive resistance. I realized that I had invested huge amounts of emotional energy into food and eating — feelings of desperation, anxiety, guilt, and shame. I also realized that I didn't ever truly enjoy any of the food I ate, that I was eating to escape.

After lots and lots of reflection, I realized that food was just food and that eating something unhealthy wasn't the end of the world. I decided to start choosing what I would eat based solely on what I wanted in that moment, which was life-changing for me. To actually care enough for myself to choose to eat something that I would enjoy without any thought to what I would look like later.

An amazing thing happened once I adopted this new mentality. Before, I had restricted myself so severely that I pushed myself into bingeing on things like cheeseburgers, fries, chips, and chocolate. But now that I was no longer depriving myself and allowing myself to eat whatever I wanted, the foods I chose to eat changed radically — and the way I ate did, too.

I quit buying prepackaged meals and started cooking for myself. I read cooking magazines and browsed cookbooks for meal ideas. I started eating new foods to see what else I might like. I started cooking for myself more and using more fresh vegetables and different types of grains to make healthier, nutrient-dense meals. I ate out far less often.

Just the act of choosing to do something positive for myself made me feel so much more confident and in control that it spurred me on to make even more changes.

I kept adding more healthy foods to what I usually ate. If I was making pasta, I added more fresh vegetables. Gradually, I began using more vegetables and less pasta. I began drinking a lot more water, which eventually displaced the diet drinks I was used to drinking. I started making fresh fruit and vegetable smoothies for breakfast, rather than skipping breakfast altogether.

I started feeling healthier, lighter, and more energized. Some of this, obviously, had to do with the changes in my diet. But mostly it had to do with my attitude toward eating and most especially toward myself. Once I took the pressure off myself to only eat certain things and avoid others, food became less scary. And once I started to be nice to myself and not judge myself so harshly, the feeling of wanting to binge started to subside.

The gradual changes I made also involved exercise. I ran track in high school, so I took up running again. My first time trying, I remember I could barely get to the end of the block without stopping. So, I stopped and walked, without mentally berating myself. Pretty soon, I had gotten up to a mile. Then I was doing two miles, the most I had ever run. Then I signed up for a 5K and did that.

It was so wonderful having a goal that had nothing to do with what I looked like or how much I weighed. After doing the 5K, I signed up for a 10K, which I also did. Six miles was a long way to me at that time. Finishing that race felt like a huge accomplishment. Then, my brother, who is a big runner, convinced me to sign up for a half marathon. He flew in from Los Angeles, where he was living, to run it with me in Atlanta. Of course, after doing the half, I knew I had to do a full marathon. So, in 1997, I trained for and ran the Los Angeles marathon.

I spent hours and hours training for that event, and on those eternal long runs, out in the middle of nowhere, I had plenty of time to reflect on how far I had come. The feeling I had from setting all these smaller goals, leading to larger and larger ones, and achieving them, was beyond empowering. Training for those races helped me to shift my focus from what I looked like to what I was able to do. My ability to complete an entire marathon — which a few years before would have seemed inconceivable — showed me what I was capable of, not just physically but also mentally.

And as I learned to shift my focus from what I looked like to what I could do, my body miraculously started to change. As I began achieving these goals, the way I thought of myself also radically changed. Whereas before my primary identity was as a girl who was always on a diet, it gradually changed into "runner" and then "marathon runner." I started to see that as I changed how I saw myself, I changed how I talked to myself. And then my "self" actually changed.

While I was training for the marathon, I started experimenting with the foods that I ate to see if adding or eliminating certain foods changed how I felt while I was running. Without any kind of planning, I gradually became a vegetarian, which was another positive distinction I could make about myself. I started reading more about nutrition and health to understand how my body worked and how the foods I ate affected me biologically.

Over the next few years, I ran a few more marathons and also gathered the courage to quit a job I hated to move to France for a year. I packed an extra suitcase full of books about nutrition and health to read and study while I was there.

When I got back home, I got another job and signed up for a nutrition class at a local university, which I attended after work. It was becoming obvious to me that my passion was anything involving nutrition, health, and learning about how to live a healthy life. So, I quit my job (again), went back to school full-time, and became a registered dietitian in 2005.

Today, I look and feel like a completely different person than I just described. Yes, my body dramatically changed, but most of all, my outlook on my life and how I see myself changed. I let go of the resistance I had toward eating and toward my body and replaced it with acceptance and a willingness to start where I was and go forward, one step at a time. I learned how to make small, manageable changes over time, which was a learning experience that gave me the confidence to make other, more challenging changes.

I learned how to take responsibility for my health, rather than putting all my hopes into a diet that was destined to fail in the long run. I shifted my perspective from the short-term "lose weight by this date" mentality and replaced with a long-term outlook that this is my lifetime journey. I learned to look at myself from the inside out rather than from the outside in, which was the catalyst for real change. I learned to love myself — which is what allowed me to effortlessly change the body I had previously so desperately hated.

None of this happened overnight. It was a long process, filled with a lot of trial and error. I had to be patient with myself and to repeatedly silence that critical inner voice that told me how far I still had to go. I had to constantly remind myself that I was after progress, not perfection. A lot of the habits I tried changing were easy to change; others were difficult. However, the process was and still is a journey, and it's one I'm committed to and that I'm having fun on.

My early conditioning with food and eating is not completely erased. It's still there, but it has faded dramatically and is now overlaid with a new conditioning — conditioning that I deliberately

86

chose rather than subconsciously developed. I still to this day struggle, and I still have days when I look in the mirror and don't like what I see.

But the difference now is that I know that my body looks the way it does as a direct result of the actions I take consistently. It isn't a reflection of who I am — only of what I do. And I know that what I have to offer goes far beyond what I see in my mirror. But best of all, now I know what I'm capable of. I know I can set goals that seem out of reach and actually achieve them. And I know that there's no limit to what I can do.

I used to think that having the body I always wanted would make me happy and that if I had it my life would be complete. Now I see clearly that the reason that body eluded me for so long was because I wasn't happy, nor was I complete. Once I made the decision to change those inner things, the body I always wanted finally began to emerge.

I've given you such an intimate account of what I went through, because I want you to know beyond a shadow of a doubt that if someone like me can do all of this, you can, too.

Most of all, I want you to know that your life is too valuable for you to waste it trying to lose weight. You don't have to spend one more minute on a diet, hating your body and agonizing about what you look like.

Make the decision right now that you're going to just stop — all of it. Take a deep breath, accept where you are, and get ready to make real changes.

Get ready for the transformation that comes with choosing to love and care for yourself and taking responsibility for your life. Get ready for the transformation that comes with believing that you're capable of more and acting on that belief.

And get ready to wake up one day and realize that you should have dreamed even bigger — that there's no limit to what you can do.

Changing Your Thoughts

Change your thoughts, and you change your world.
— Norman Vincent Peale

Y ou are in a constant conversation with yourself — all day, every day. However, you're probably not consciously aware of it.

You may know intellectually that this inner conversation exists, but unless you're paying close attention, it's hard to spot. That's because you're so used to hearing it that it's become like white noise.

The problem about not noticing it is that these inner conversations frequently veer off into dangerous territory. At best, some of them are merely unproductive — but at worst they can be downright destructive.

You have to identify and change the negative back-and-forth you have with yourself if you want to be successful at anything in life. All of us have a critical inner voice, but if you want to succeed at anything you do — be it running a company or running your home — you have to change that negative voice into something far different (or at least turn the volume down).

The conversations you have with yourself, if they go on long enough, eventually establish beliefs. And a set of beliefs becomes an identity. So, if you don't learn to spot the negative voice in your head and change it, you'll eventually become someone you don't want to be. You'll create an identity for yourself that limits you and keeps you from living the life you deserve to live.

And what's worse, you'll subconsciously believe that this identity is who you really are . . . when the reality is, it's solely based on the lies you tell yourself.

If you don't shut that voice down, you'll absorb it and gradually, over time, accept it as fact. Eventually an identity forms, and it won't be anything close to the real you.

Unfortunately, in some cases the identity takes over, and that person then continues act in ways that back up that identity — sometimes for years. And what you have then is a life not fully lived.

It's imperative that you spot that critical voice, and it's vital that you challenge it and change it.

If that voice continues long enough, you start believing that the major accomplishments of others aren't for someone like you, and you think things like "I could never do that" when you see other people achieve big goals. As a result, you won't try new things — you hold yourself back. And this is how you end up spending the majority of your days obsessing about what you look like and wasting your life trying to lose weight.

If you don't learn how to spot that voice and challenge it, you'll keep yourself stuck. And not only will you not lose weight — you never get a chance to live anywhere close to your fullest potential.

So now let's talk about the specific ways that negative voice manifests as it relates to food and eating and how to put a stop to it.

The way you talk to yourself

As it relates to food, eating, dieting, and body image, your critical inner voice tells you things like you're weak and have no willpower when you try not to eat and eventually give in. When you don't stick to a diet, the voice will tell you you're a failure. When you look in the mirror and see the extra weight, the voice will tell you you're disgusting, fat, and unattractive. I'm certain that if you've struggled with your weight, you've been hearing things like this for years, right?

And I'm also certain that you've accepted these things as fact. If you believe these things about yourself, it's nearly impossible to make positive changes. But if you step back objectively and see what's really going on, you can dismantle the entire conversation and change it.

So, when it comes to eating, here are the two most problematic issues: 1) you feel like you're out of control and 2) you feel shame at being out of control. Both of these feelings arise from your thoughts.

Remember, you've trained yourself to eat to make yourself feel better. And when you eat to make yourself feel better, you eat *until* you feel better — which means you eat too fast and you overeat (in other words, you binge eat).

There are specific thoughts that lead you to a binge eating episode, and they're different for every person because every person has a unique life experience. Some of them are in response to environmental triggers, which we'll talk more about later.

However, even though everyone's thoughts are unique, they all have a similar theme: they all stem from a feeling of being out of control.

Feeling out of control

Even though a binge-eating episode feels reflexive and automatic, it's preceded with thoughts that create anxiety or some kind of stress or discomfort. And these may not necessarily be related to food.

The feelings that push you to go looking for something to shove down are preceded by thoughts of not being able to handle whatever it is that's coming your way and an urge to relieve the discomfort you feel because of it.

In other words, a binge is a result of you not taking control of something that's happening in your life, whether it's from the past or it's happening right in the moment, and the negative feelings that result both from the event and your feeling of being unable to control it or handle it.

I'll use myself as an example. As I mentioned previously, I grew up feeling isolated and alone, even though I was surrounded by people. My overall thought was that something was wrong with me. In fact, I had a constant question in the back of my mind: *What is wrong with me?*

It was this nagging thought that isolated me from the people around me and made me feel tremendously lonely. So, I filled myself up with food. I was ashamed at my eating — how much I ate and how fast I ate it. I was ashamed of my seeming inability to control myself. And I isolated myself even more by eating alone.

I didn't have the life skills or the perspective to handle my feelings of isolation, and I felt powerless to change it. (And I also didn't know then that thinking there was something wrong with me wasn't a unique thought in the mind of a pre-teen girl.)

But I had established my emotional eating at that point and then used food to fill myself up for years afterward whenever I encountered situations where I didn't think I fit in or felt incapable of controlling what was happening.

So, an event like going away to college and having no set schedule or structure to tell me how to "be" was overwhelmingly stressful for me. I felt, quite literally, out of control. And because I felt incapable of dealing with this new world I was living in, I went to my dorm room alone and did what I always had done when I felt out of control: I ate. And the fact that I was binge eating made me feel even more out of control.

Feeling out of control in my environment was nothing compared to the loss of control I had around food. I felt tremendous, overpowering shame at the way I ate and my seeming inability to control it. And I felt even more shame at the way I looked as a result of my lack of control.

And ultimately, my inner critic put me in a shame/binge spiral I felt powerless to escape.

Your inner critic

We all have an inner critic, and there are different hypotheses as to why we have one and how it develops. One possible explanation is that we internalize the messages of authority figures who disciplined us as children and gave us the message that we should stay safe and not do anything to jeopardize that safety.

But when "Don't play in the street" is no longer necessary, as an adult you hear things like, "You don't belong here," "You never do anything right," "You look horrible," or "Why can't you just stop eating?"

The important thing to remember is that your inner critic isn't the real you. But the more you listen to it, the more you believe that it is — and then act on the false identity your inner critic has constructed for you.

So, the thoughts aren't you, but they are responsible for the actions you take. The problem is, when you do things you don't want to — like binge eat — instead of realizing that these behaviors come from your thoughts, you shame yourself for them.

The good news is that thoughts can be changed. You can systematically overhaul your thoughts. But to do this you have to notice them. You have to consciously become aware of them.

The most important thing to get at this point is that changing your thoughts is absolutely critical when it comes to changing your habits. Your habits, although they seem automatic, are entirely driven by

93

your thoughts. But right now, you're going straight from engaging in these habits to shaming yourself for them.

If you learn how to spot the thoughts that lead you to the binge then become aware of the thoughts you have both during the binge and after the binge, you can change those thoughts.

And when you start changing the thoughts, you start changing the behavior, which means you change the habit.

The way you see yourself

How you talk to yourself drives how you see yourself, and this creates your identity.

The reason identity is so important is that you live to the identity you've created for yourself. So, if you see yourself in a limited way, you're going to live a small life, one that's way short of your true potential.

If you spend your time constantly trying to lose weight, it's partly because you see yourself in this limited way. And seeing yourself in a limited way keeps you living a small life — which means you waste a huge chunk of your time trying to lose weight. It's a cycle.

One issue is that you probably don't have a true, strong identity. Instead, as is usually the case with the women I work with, you're probably living a series of roles and seeing yourself through the lens of those roles.

First off, roles can't exist without other people involved. So, when you live out a role, you're living according to what other people expect of you instead of for yourself and what you want. A role is about other people — an identity is about you.

Constantly trying to lose weight is a natural extension of living like this, because what's behind wanting to lose weight is a desire to look a certain way for other people and to fit into a culture that beats it into us that all we ultimately have to offer is our looks.

94

If you can relate to this, then it's likely that you're defining yourself based on a series of roles. This keeps you doing and doing to fit the roles, rather than living in a strong, confident way because of a positive identity you've created for yourself.

Living from a strong sense of self influences you to engage in positive, creative activities that support the identity — activities like eating healthy and exercising — and that naturally have all kinds of positive outcomes — like clear skin, quality sleep, and a lean, toned body.

Roles are about doing, whereas an identity is about being — and then the "doing" flows naturally from it. When you live according to a role, it's about actions you take. But if you live according to an identity, it's about who you are, and the actions follow naturally.

So, for example, I am a mom — "mom" is my role. However, my identity is that I'm a guide and a role model for two human beings. And my actions reflect the difference between these two things.

When I act from a place of being a mom, I think of driving them to school, feeding them, and caring for them, all of which are important. But when I think of myself as a guide, my motivations become different — and then so do my actions. When I act from my identity, I think of teaching them to eat healthy, to be kind and empathetic, to try new things. And I do all of this by modeling those things to them, because of it being an identity rather than a role.

Once my kids are grown, I'm no longer a mom. Obviously, I'll always be "Mom" to my daughters, but the *role* of mom — cleaning up after them, feeding them, putting on Band-Aids, and attending their recitals — is over when they leave the nest. Roles have an expiration date. Identities don't. I will never stop being a guide, teacher, and role model to them.

Also, my identity as a guide means I'm living from an expansive place where the actions I take strengthen me as a woman and a human being. Whereas doing mostly benefits them, being means I also benefit.

Your identity is the most powerful motivating force behind what you do. So, if your identity is based on roles you play — I'm a mom, I'm a volunteer, I'm a wife, I'm an employee — you're going to live in a smaller way.

Don't get me wrong: roles are important and give you a sense of purpose and worth. They are valuable. But the thing about roles is that they revolve around other people and what you do for them, and the worth you derive from performing them is based on how those people perceive you to have performed.

If they think you did a good job and you lived up to their expectations, everything's great. But if you don't — even if you gave it your all — your self-esteem suffers. If you're living out your roles without a strong identity, your self-worth is at the mercy of others.

But when you start choosing an identity for yourself, your self-worth is determined by you and only you. So, when you stumble and fall, you didn't let anyone down. You get to choose to learn from it and grow, and it doesn't matter what anyone else thinks. When you have your own identity, there is no limit to how you define it or what you can do.

An identity has tremendous energy behind it, because at its core, an identity is you putting your power out into the universe and saying, "This is who I am." And claiming your inner power means you're taking responsibility for yourself, your actions, and where you are right now. When you have a strong sense of self, that means you can problem-solve, make changes, and get things done. When you have a strong sense of self, you're not concerned with what other people think of you — especially if their opinion has to do with what you look like.

Spending all your time constantly trying to lose weight to meet an external expectation of what you should look like is the opposite of developing a strong sense of self and claiming your internal power.

Wrapping up your worth in what you look like in a bathing suit, how much cellulite you have on the back of your legs, and how your arms look in a sleeveless shirt is confidence-draining and soul-destroying. That's because you're living according to other people's perception of you.

When your existence involves what other people think of you — especially if it's because of how you look — you can't be the strong, confident woman you were meant to be. And a strong, confident woman doesn't desperately try to diet weight off her body. A strong, confident woman with a firmly established identity takes care of herself and her body, because she feels good about herself.

Having a strong identity and seeing yourself in a more powerful way takes you out of the binge/gain/diet/fail cycle. Expressing your internal power via a strong identity means that every action you take from that place will naturally support a healthy mind and a healthy body. You won't have to try "not to" do certain things. You naturally won't do unhealthy things — you'll naturally have healthy habits that mean you take the right actions automatically.

So, for example, a vegetarian doesn't have to try not to eat meat, and she also naturally eats tons of fruits and vegetables. A marathon runner doesn't have to try not to skip a workout, and she also effortlessly gets tons of exercise. An actress doesn't have to try not to binge eat, and she naturally eats slowly and mindfully. A CEO doesn't have to force herself to go to work, and she naturally gets there on time (or earlier). These are all identities.

So how do you develop an identity? You set a larger goal for yourself. Anyone who dares to set a bigger goal has already taken the first step in creating an identity. Choosing a goal, saying "I'm going to do this," and then making a plan to do it sparks belief in yourself.

Then as you work steadily toward achieving that goal, getting small wins along the way and building your confidence, a new identity starts to take shape.

We'll talk about having a larger goal and exactly how to set it and achieve it a little later. But for now, there are some other tactics you can use to establish a strong, powerful identity for yourself.

But first let's look at the process for changing how you think.

Change how you talk to yourself

Your inner critic will passively brainwash you into believing that you're lazy, out of control, and have no willpower if you don't develop awareness about what's really going on. You can't feel empowered to make changes when you feel this way about yourself, and this is exactly why so many people stay stuck for so long.

They get in a cycle of blame and shame instead of objectively seeing what's happening. So, the first step is to recognize that there's a reason you're engaging in these habits. And, no, it's not because you're out of control — it's because of your thoughts.

You have specific thoughts around food and eating that create your eating habits. And you have thoughts that push you to engage in these habits, thoughts while you're engaging in them, and thoughts that occur after you do.

Identifying each of these thoughts, analyzing them, and deliberately altering them is half of the equation that will help eliminate the habit (the other being making microchanges to the habit, which we'll cover in the next chapter).

Habits feel automatic because you've trained yourself to engage in them for so long. But there are triggers that start an avalanche of negative thoughts that push you into those habits, and there are associations you make when you engage in them that keep them entrenched.

Let's look at an example. You're stressed out because your kids are fighting and the house is a mess, so you grab a bag of chips out of the pantry, lock yourself in your bedroom, and shove them down until you feel better.

You engage in a habit like this in what feels like a split second. One minute you're in the living room picking toys up off the floor, and the next you're in your bedroom with your hand in a bag of chips. But if you look closely at this habit, you'll see there's a lot going on under the surface.

First you have an environmental trigger: stress and overwhelm. Your kids are fighting, which is stressful, and your house is a mess, which makes you feel overwhelmed and even more stressed.

These feelings then cause thoughts like, "I do everything around here with no help" or "No one appreciates anything I do" or "I'm so sick of hearing these kids fight all the time." These thoughts then push you to grab the chips, an action that also has associated thoughts: "I'm dying for some chips" or "I need to eat something." Then your decision to go off by yourself is backed up with thoughts: "I just want to be alone" or "I never get a moment's peace." Then you binge eat until the feeling of being overwhelmed subsides, which it does because of the thoughts you're thinking: "These are so good" or "Now I feel better."

Environmental triggers cause thoughts that push you into bad habits, and then you make positive associations with these habits that keep you from changing them. You're associating escaping the chaos and going off alone in your room to binge eat potato chips with feeling better. And all of these actions are backed up with thoughts — you're just not noticing it.

I cannot stress this enough: Your thoughts are a powerful invisible force that pushes you to make decisions almost instantaneously. And then when you give in to a binge, your inner critic shames you for doing it. It all goes back to your thoughts.

Don't forget that feeling out of control — meaning incapable of dealing with what's going on inside you or around you — is the common denominator in emotional eating. You've trained yourself to use food to deal with feelings like pain, frustration, anger, or loneliness. And if you feel these things for an extended period, it's because you're not taking action to deal with them. In other words, you're being powerless and not taking control.

Once you deconstruct a habit like bingeing, you have a ton of options to work with. (Isn't that good news? You don't have to just try to quit binge eating Doritos.) You have the environmental triggers (kids, a messy house), you have the emotional triggers (stress, overwhelm), and you have the thoughts (before, during, and after the habit).

So, the first and most obvious place to start is managing the environmental trigger. You can do things like hire a housekeeper to help you keep your house clean or hire a babysitter a few hours a day to help you with your kids.

The next step is to manage how you respond to your environment. It takes practice to manage your emotions, and it starts with managing your thoughts. You have to teach yourself to be proactive rather than reactive.

Remove yourself from the environment and do something proactive — like breathe deeply, walk around the block, or call a friend — rather than reacting and eating something.

Doing any of these first three things gives you an opportunity to work through your thoughts and feelings. Figure out exactly what you're thinking and what your inner conversation is. Make a constructive plan to change the environmental stressors that are occurring. It's true that if you can't change what's happening, you can at least change how you respond to it.

But it takes practice to go from binge eating to effectively managing your circumstances and your reactions to them. Don't forget you've trained yourself for years to respond to any kind of stress with food.

So, if you find yourself in the middle of a binge — don't worry. This is your opportunity to figure out what you're thinking and then work on changing those thoughts.

What did you think about immediately before you grabbed the chips? If it was, "I just want some chips," you could rephrase it as a question: "Do I really want some chips?" If your thought was "I just want to be alone," you could change that to "I just need some space," which isn't as forceful and decreases the impulse to binge.

Even if you find yourself alone in your room with a bag of chips, you have a chance to make progress. If you're thinking "These are so good," you could rephrase that as a question: "Are these really good?" And instead of "Now I feel better," you could ask "How does eating this really make me feel?" Or even better, "What would actually make me feel better?"

After the binge, if you're thinking "Why did I just do that? I am so disgusting. Why can't I just stop eating?" answer the first question. Why did you grab a bag of chips and start eating? Answers: "I'm completely overwhelmed with everything I have to do around here," "I need some help with the kids, and it's worse in the afternoon," or "I didn't get enough sleep last night, and I'm exhausted." Now you can manage those stressors.

And are you really "disgusting"? No. Do you *feel* disgusting? Maybe. But now that changes the narrative. And "Why can't I just stop eating?" could be changed to "Why do I feel like I can't stop?"

I hope you can see from this one example how much progress you can make by simply becoming aware of your thoughts and how they're there behind the scenes practically pushing you into that habit.

You can take any bad habit and analyze it carefully to see what thoughts are behind it. And then you can systematically work on changing any one of those thoughts to start the process of changing the habit.

How to do it

Now let's break the process down into basic steps. The four steps in changing your thoughts are:

1. Develop awareness
2. Identify thoughts and triggers
3. Challenge and change the thoughts
4. Practice

Before we look at each step, the first thing I want you to do is get a journal. I can hear you protesting already. I know that you're resisting this step, but you can't change your thoughts just by noticing a few of them here and there and trying to change them in your mind. It won't work. And I know that journaling is not something you're excited about doing.

How do I know this? Because I used to resist it, too. It's sort of like meditating. It feels hard because it requires being calm and still, finding the time to do it, and doing it in the midst of a chaotic life that feels like everything is conspiring against you to prevent you from doing it. Who feels like they have the luxury of sitting down with a journal and writing down their thoughts when they have twenty loads of laundry and can barely find time to get dressed?

Well, you do. And if you don't think you have the time, you have to make the time. And isn't it worth it to spend a little time now getting to the root of the problem rather than waste your entire life dieting?

The main reason people resist journaling — or at least the reason I did — is that there's no formula for doing it. Since there aren't any directions, you'll be wondering if you're doing it right or not.

There is no right or wrong way. Even if there's a day where all you write is one sentence, that's okay. And if you have to write down a thought while you're at a traffic light on your morning commute or while you're listening to your kids scream, that's good enough. You don't have to be sitting in a perfectly clean house with candles lit and soft music playing — in fact, I expect you to not be in that space most of the time. (But if you are, that's totally fabulous, and good for you!)

I'm about to give you a basic structure to follow to make it easier, but please do not skip this critical step. You don't have to be perfect, and if you miss a few days just jump right back in. But do it! There's so much evidence that writing things down makes you far more likely to remember them, and if you're writing down goals that you'll achieve them (more on that later).

So put this book down right now, go to your favorite stationery store, and buy yourself a beautiful brand-new journal. By taking this one simple step, you're signaling your brain that you're committed and now taking action, which gives you tremendous confidence.

Step 1: Develop awareness

You can't be aware of something unless you stop and look, recognize it there in front of you, and call it what it is. It sounds obvious, but even the actual things you look at around you start to become invisible after a while.

Think about it. You could tell me what kind of furniture you have in your living room, but could you describe the paintings on your walls, the molding that's around your ceiling, or the books on your bookshelf? Probably not, because you're so used to seeing them that you aren't really aware of them.

Your thoughts are no different. To become aware, you have to stop, focus consciously, notice, and process. If you had to describe a painting in your bedroom, you need to stop in front of it, focus on it, notice the individual elements, and name them to tell someone about them.

Whenever you feel yourself impulsively doing something or feel like you're about to, stop for a minute. Stop what you're doing physically, and pay attention to the chatter in your head. Be fully present and notice the thoughts. Mentally step back from your thoughts, and see them separately from yourself. Seeing them as not being "you" will really help you be objective and get a sense of control. Your thoughts are in control of you if you're not aware of them; once you become aware of what they are, you control them.

When you do this, you'll be really surprised at how many thoughts you're having at once. Once you can identify them, process the tone of the thoughts. Do you feel out of control? Do you feel like you're telling yourself the wrong story about who you are? Do you see how you might be creating even more stress with the thoughts? Do you feel good, bad, happy, afraid, joyful, panicky, frustrated, irritated, overwhelmed, energized, exhausted?

Being aware and conscious shows you that what seem to be urges and impulses are actually a flood of thoughts rushing by that you have total control over.

Step 2: Identify thoughts and triggers

There are two kinds of triggers that start a cascade of thoughts: environmental and emotional.

As we saw in the example I just gave, there are usually many environmental triggers involved in binge eating or destructive eating habits. They're fairly easy to identify, because what they have in common is that they typically create stress, frustration, or overwhelm.

Your house looks like a bomb went off, your kids are fighting, you have way too many things on your to-do list, you're tired and irritated because you didn't sleep last night, you missed your morning workout, you spilled red wine on the carpet. (Maybe all of the above.)

Once you identify these triggers, you can manage them or avoid them altogether. Ask your husband and kids to pitch in with the housekeeping. Get a housekeeper once a month. Get an afternoon sitter once a week. Ask your husband to come home early a few nights a week. Eliminate some of the things on your to-do list. RSVP no. Go to bed earlier. Set your alarm earlier. Don't drink red wine (just kidding).

An important side note here is that we as women are always doing things for everyone else and hardly ever for ourselves. So, for the list above, I would take it one step further. If you get a sitter for your kids, don't run errands — go get a manicure. If you go to bed earlier, light a candle first and have some relaxation time to unwind. If you get up earlier, don't just jump into your day — read something inspiring while you have coffee. Give yourself a half hour each day to do absolutely nothing.

A lot of the stress I used to feel was because I was trying to do absolutely everything and then telling myself how no one helped me or appreciated me and on and on — and then I never asked for help or took some of the pointless things off my list. Don't be a martyr. Don't try to do everything by yourself. And if no one truly appreciates you, then you walk out the door, go do something you love, and appreciate yourself!

Now let's look at emotional triggers. Feeling depressed, angry, sad, helpless, and bored are all binge-eating triggers. Emotional triggers are usually preceded by environmental triggers, so you can also manage your external environment to prevent these emotions from coming up.

If you feel depressed or sad, figure out what's causing it. Do you feel lonely because you live by yourself and spend a ton of time alone? Call a friend and go shopping or have coffee. If you feel angry because of a relationship issue or because of something that happened in your past, make an appointment to see a therapist. (The best thing I have ever done for myself.) If you're bored in your down time, instead of sitting in front of the television do something productive. Go for a walk or do a home-improvement project.

If you can deal with the emotional and environmental triggers on the front end, you can avoid a lot of the thoughts that arise that push you into binge eating.

So, once you've got a handle on these triggers, you need to identify the thoughts and associations you're making before you binge, while you binge, and after you binge. They're different for everyone, so you have to identify yours.

Before the binge, you're may be thinking things like, "I am so sick of this," "I just need to eat something," "I want some chocolate," or "I never do anything right."

During the binge you may be thinking, "This is so delicious" or "I feel so much better." You're making positive associations with eating, which reinforces using food as a reward. Thoughts like "I deserve this" or "I've been so good all day" are indicators that you're rewarding yourself with food. If you're an emotional eater, you likely get into a zoned-out state while you're eating. Pull yourself out of this, and notice the thoughts you're having.

Notice where and when you binge. Do you binge in front of the television or computer? Do you go off alone? Do you binge in the afternoon or late at night? If it feels good to sit in front of your computer and binge, if it feels good to get away from everyone and binge, or if it feels good late afternoon when you've been on the go all day to binge as your reward for working so hard, these are all opportunities to make changes.

The thoughts you have after a binge are where you can make the most progress. This is where the voice of your inner critic is on full blast, telling you how weak and worthless you are, how out of control you are, and how disgusting you look. It's shocking to see how mean you are to yourself once you start identifying what your inner critic says.

Identifying thoughts and triggers is dependent on awareness, so the first two steps go hand-in-hand. Once you start paying attention and spotting these destructive thoughts, you're ready for step three: changing them.

Step 3: Challenge and change the thoughts

Now that you're really focusing in on your thoughts and identifying them, it's time to change them.

The way you do this is to challenge them by asking questions until you get to something objective or some kind of tactic you can use — instead of being stuck in a shame spiral and feeling helpless and out of control.

But, again, you can't do this just in your mind — you have to write the thoughts down on paper. I know it's tempting to skip this important step, but please don't! This is where you'll really make progress, because seeing your thoughts in black and white shows you just how much you're sabotaging yourself and how much room for improvement there is. And by writing the thoughts down, you have a much better chance of successfully changing them than if you try to do it mentally.

What you want to do is have your journal with you at all times. This is easy when you're at home, but make sure to take it with you when you're out at dinner, when you're traveling, when you're at work — even when you're running errands or sitting in the carpool line. Negative, self-defeating, and destructive thoughts that are driving all your bad habits occur at any point throughout the day, not just when you're eating.

So, whenever a thought comes up that may be preventing you from making progress, write it down. Thoughts about how you've got to try not to eat so much today, thoughts about how you dread something, thoughts about how fat you feel or how gross you think you look, thoughts about how "over it" you are — nothing is irrelevant. And if you're not somewhere where it's easy or feasible to pull out your journal, make the best mental notes you can and then write them down as soon as possible.

Obviously, you really want to home in on what you're thinking about just before you eat, while you're eating, and after you eat. Ideally, you should try to be present while you're eating, but if you find yourself in an out-of-control binge at some point, don't worry. As you start changing your thoughts and your habits, these will occur less frequently and with less intensity.

Now here's where the rubber meets the road. At the end of the day (or more frequently if you can), you're going to review your thoughts and challenge them.

Here's how you do that. For every thought you've written down, you want to question it. So, for example, if you've written down "I am so disgusting," you want to ask yourself, "Am I really disgusting? If you've written down, "I am so sick of doing everything myself," you want to ask yourself, "Why do I feel this way?" If you've written "I need to eat something," you want to ask, "Why do I need to eat something?"

Your ultimate goal is to keep asking questions until you get to the root of what's really going on and find the objective truth behind it. So, let's use the example "I need to eat something." Here's what your questioning process might look like:

I need to eat something.
Why do you need to eat something?
Because I'm totally stressed out and it would make me feel better.
Why do you feel stressed?

Because the house is a mess, and I don't feel like cleaning it, and I'm tired of doing everything myself.

How can you change this? What could you do to make these things easier?

I could have the kids clean up their rooms themselves, I could take a break from cleaning and sit outside instead, and I could talk to my husband about how overwhelmed I feel.

Why would eating make you feel better?

Because it feels good to zone out and binge.

What happens after you binge?

I feel awful and hate myself for doing it.

Is the binge worth it if you're going to feel like this when it's over?

No.

What else could you do to make yourself feel better?

I could go outside and get away from the chaos for ten minutes, I could take a walk, I could call a friend.

Now you have something to work with. You can see how your thoughts are pushing you to binge, and now that you know what they are and have questioned them, you can also see that what you're saying to yourself isn't necessarily true. You also now have alternatives to bingeing that you can use.

Most importantly, you've taken the emotion and intensity out of it, and you feel more calm and in control. You're not just at the mercy of your impulse to eat whenever things are stressful. And now you can easily see that it's not just because you can't stick to anything or have no willpower — what you're thinking is actually pushing you to eat.

Let's use another example:

I am so disgusting.

109

Are you really disgusting?
No, but I feel disgusting.
Why do you feel this way?
Because my fat is hanging over my jeans, and I'm exhausted from sucking my stomach in all the time.
What could you do to feel differently?
I could wear something that isn't skintight, and I could work on standing naturally without sucking my stomach in.

I'm not suggesting here that you should start ordering clothes in a size up and stop caring, of course. But getting rid of resistance immediately increases your chances of success, and loving yourself where you are now is critical to move forward. Also, there's a big difference between *being* disgusting and *feeling* disgusting.

Here's another example from my life. One of the worst habits I needed to change was eating too fast, which usually happened when I was in front of the television or the computer. (Remember how I taught myself to do this early on?)

There were times when all of my best-laid plans to make a healthy meal and sit quietly at the table, eating slowly and mindfully, went out the window. Like when my kids want to order pizza and watch a movie with me, for example.

My inner argument would start with "Ugh. You're supposed to have a salad." Then "But you can't just never eat pizza again," "You can't miss this time with the girls," and "You can make up for it tomorrow." And then I would sit in front of the television with my daughters and zone out while I scarfed down three pieces of pizza.

Then of course I would be mad at myself for not "sticking" to my healthy plan, and I would tell myself how gross I was for doing that and that nothing was ever going to change.

But when I challenged these thoughts, here's what happened:

You can't just never eat pizza again.
No, but can you eat it differently?
Yes.
How could you do that?
Get one slice, cut it into pieces, and eat more slowly; add some
fruit on the side; take sips of water in between bites.

You can't miss this time with the girls.
Do you have to?
No.
How could you enjoy it and also be healthy?
[Take the steps above], and also feel good that you're showing
your girls how to eat in a healthy way.

You can make up for it tomorrow.
Make up for what?
Enjoying a few slices of pizza.
What's enjoyable about it?
The feeling I get from shoving it down and not having to be
"good."
How do you feel after you do this?
Like crap.
Is there a way to enjoy it without shoving it down?
Yes, I could [take the steps above].

I saw from taking the whole conversation apart how I was
equating shoving down food with feeling good and how I was
labeling some foods as "good" or "bad" — all of which kept fueling
my emotional eating. By doing this I was able to dial down the drama
and see everything more rationally. I felt more in control by not
making it an either/or, all-or-nothing scenario: either I eat a salad or I

binge on pizza. I gave myself space to enjoy a less-than-healthy meal and watch a movie with my kids. And I didn't have to make up for anything the next day and keep starting over with all the craziness: "Tomorrow I'll be good."

By continuing your question-and-answer process until you get to an objective truth, you get rid of all the emotion and can calmly come up with solutions and take control.

Once you've challenged the thoughts, it's time to change them. For every thought you have, pick the three to five that feel the most destructive or that you suspect may be holding you back the most.

Out to the side of each thought, re-write the thought in its more accurate or less-extreme form, and turn it into something that makes you feel in control instead of helpless. Here are some examples:

I need to eat something.
I can eat something if I choose to.

Why can't I just lose weight?
Losing weight isn't complicated, and I can do it if I decide to.

I am so disgusting.
I feel heavy and bloated.

Why does this always happen to me?
Nothing happens to me. I make things happen.

This candy is delicious.
This candy tastes good and I'm choosing to eat it, but it's not fueling my body.

I need some chocolate.

I feel like I want something sweet.

I hate working out.
Working out is challenging, but I do it because it makes me stronger.

You can hopefully see from these examples how these slight modifications take the intensity out of the statements and change you from a victim to being in charge. You can take this as far as you want — have fun with it! The point is to change your habitual thoughts into statements that take the shame and powerlessness out of your usual thoughts.

It's important that you write the new statements down on paper and tweak them until they resonate with you. Once you have them down, you're going to practice them.

Step 4: Practice

When practicing your newly changed thoughts, there are some effective strategies you can use to help cement them into your subconscious.

Before we get to them, it's helpful to start with only one or two at a time. Of the several that you've identified that most hold you back, pick two of them and focus on those until you've got them down. Here are some additional tactics that will make them even more powerful.

1. Eliminate exaggerated language. You did this in step one of changing the thought, but it's really important to tone down the language. The reason is that using exaggerated language creates unnecessary urgency and feelings of desperation and not being in control.

When you use words like *hate, never, always,* and *can't,* it makes you feel like you've gone past the point of no return and there's no way back. This equals powerlessness.

It also makes things seem way more dramatic than they are. After all, what we're dealing with here is simply needing to change your eating habits and patterns. It's not the end of the world, and it's not a problem that can't be solved.

Choose more balanced language. Change hate to "not my favorite," change never and always to "sometimes," change can't to "it's simple and doable." Being less exaggerated also helps you take the emotion out of it. Emotionally charged language lends itself to personal-attack statements that make you feel bad and keep you stuck.

2. Address yourself as "you." I like to call this my Inner Cheerleader. Instead of saying "I" in your mind, talk to yourself as if there's another person there. Say "you."

For example, if you're changing the thought, "I am so disgusting," and you've modified it to, "I feel bloated," take it one step farther and say, "You feel bloated right now."

There are two reasons for doing this. The first is that when you address yourself as if you're an internal coach, it's like you're having a conversation with someone. Because of this, it's natural to keep going. So, if you say to yourself, "You feel bloated right now," the follow-up might be, "and you can change that."

The second reason is that ultra-successful people do this. Success coach Brendon Burchard studied one hundred of the most successful people alive to find out what practices they have in common. One of them was addressing themselves as "you" instead of "I."

They created their own mental motivational coach, and doing this seems to be one common denominator that contributed to their massive success. So, if the world's most successful people do it, why not you?

3. Ask questions. Phrasing your new thought in the form of a question is tremendously helpful, because it puts you in problem-solving mode. To use the example above, you've turned "I am so disgusting" into "You feel bloated right now." To increase its effectiveness, you could make it, "Why do you feel bloated right now?"

That way, you naturally look for answer and therefore have to come up with one. If you ask yourself why you feel this way, you figure out what you're doing wrong. If you ask yourself why you feel bloated, the answers might be because you drank too much last night, you're bingeing on chocolate every day after lunch, or that you haven't been working out regularly.

By identifying specific causes, you will then seek out solutions. This is the complete opposite of telling yourself that you are disgusting, which is a paralyzing personal attack that keeps you stuck.

4. Create a mantra. The stories we tell ourselves have a huge impact on our results. A lot of the stories we tell are just flat-out not true, and we keep them going with thoughts that back them up.

So, to create an entirely new story, the most powerful thing you can add is a mantra that you repeat throughout the day. Create one that motivates you to action. Some examples are, "I feel vibrant and alive," "I kick ass at life," "Everything about me is truly beautiful." A few of mine are "Today is the day" and "Start before you're ready."

Contrast that with the typical things we tell ourselves: "Nothing is ever easy," "I could never do that," or "This always happens to me."

Or how about "Life's a bitch and then you die" or "There aren't enough hours in the day"?

A good, strong, positive mantra gives you confidence, creative energy, and motivation to take action. Adding a mantra supercharges your ability to transform your thinking, especially if you repeat it often.

Create one that lights your inner fire and makes you want to jump out of bed every day, ready to change your life!

Change your identity

We've covered how you talk to yourself, so now let's discuss how to change how you see yourself. It can feel hard to see yourself in a different way and live to an identity — especially if you've been living a series of roles for years on end.

When you're growing up, the sky's the limit in terms of who you can become. You had endless choices and possibilities, and everyone around you was constantly asking, "What do you want to be when you grow up?" You also had distinct phases you traveled through on your journey to adulthood: middle school, high school, college, and the years in your first job.

But once you get married and start a family, the years begin to blend together, and the phases dwindle. You become a wife and a mom — and you stay that way. And before you know it, ten years have passed and you may no longer have a true sense of who you are.

This is how it's so easy to lose yourself in a meaningless pursuit of weight loss. Your identity becomes lost as you start seeing yourself through the lens of others, and you dumb your goals down to match. You lose your voice and sense of internal power, so you start getting your worth by conforming to other people's expectations — being the perfect wife, being the perfect mom, having the perfect body.

You have to deliberately pull yourself out of this fog, where you're being brainwashed to believe that there's nothing abnormal about obsessing about how much you weigh, constantly talking about how fat you look, and wasting all your time trying to figure out what diet to go on next.

You have to wake up every day and remind yourself that none of this is normal. You have to wake up every day and retrain your brain to focus on something different. And the easiest way to shift your focus is to start seeing yourself differently — to create a new identity for yourself, in which you are powerful, in control, and filled with excitement.

This is the polar opposite of rolling out of bed, dreading another day filled with responsibilities and care-taking activities, wondering if you'll have enough willpower to stick to your diet.

It's pretty clear that a strong, powerful, self-confident woman who is on fire for life doesn't get up this way, and it's also pretty clear that as long as you keep living this way, you'll never become that strong, powerful, self-confident woman.

So, here's the tricky part. To start seeing yourself this way, you have to start acting differently. But for you to take the right actions, you have to start changing how you see yourself.

The taking action part of the equation is in setting a larger goal for yourself, which we'll get to later. For now, let's talk about creating the new identity.

How you see yourself now is powerless, not in control, and at the mercy of your circumstances. You would probably challenge me on this, but I'm talking about subconscious powerlessness.

You don't feel powerless on the surface because you've become so adept at mastering your many roles. You may be an outstanding employee, a superstar PTA president, or a true Supermom. But, again, if you're living to fulfill the expectations of other people, you're not expressing your true power, taking control over your own life, speaking with your authentic voice, and living with one hundred percent enthusiasm.

As it relates to food, eating, and losing weight, you're approaching it as if you're stuck, helpless, and paralyzed by your circumstances — all of which make you feel desperate and push you to take drastic actions like starve yourself or crash diet.

How you want to see yourself is in control and in charge of your life, full of power to make permanent changes, because you decide to make them and then follow through — without anyone telling you what to do. And how you do this is to create a stronger identity for yourself.

So, you want to develop an identity that has nothing to do with losing weight and that makes weight loss effortless. Instead of thinking of yourself as a middle-aged woman going through menopause who has a hard time losing weight, a better identity would be a triathlete who naturally takes actions that result in a lean, toned body.

Here are some strategies to use in creating a new identity:

Choose the identity. You can do this two ways. You can create something entirely new, or you can flesh out one of your current roles.

To create a totally new identity, pick something you always wanted to do — like write, paint, design jewelry, travel, or become an accountant. So, your new identity would be writer, artist, jewelry designer, world traveler, or financial planner. Obviously, pick something that gets you excited and motivated.

If you want to upgrade a role, pick one you currently have and magnify it. If you're a stockbroker, think of yourself as a wealth creator. If you're a doctor, think of yourself as a healer. If you're a mom, think of yourself as a spiritual teacher, a feminist role model, or a guide who shapes future leaders.

Think as big as you can, and don't limit yourself based on your current circumstances. If you're a mom to two teenagers and feel stretched to your limit with everything you have to do, don't let that stop you from allowing yourself to dream a little bit. There's no reason to keep something that's totally possible for you from entering your consciousness and becoming a reality just because you have a to-do list a mile long. (This is the whole point, by the way!)

And you don't have to limit yourself to just one identity. I think of myself as a writer, a feminist role model to my daughters, a world traveler, a marathon runner, and a vegetarian. But one is all you need to get started!

Flesh it out on paper. Write down the traits or habits this kind of person has. If you want to be an artist, you would be creative, inspired, prolific, focused, or fulfilled. If you want to be a feminist role model, you would be courageous, passionate, outspoken, motivated to action, and a rule-breaker. If you want to be a world traveler, you would be investigative, eager to learn, a planner, open-minded, and adventurous.

Write down anything and everything you can think of that's related to the identity. What you would wear (are you a doctor in a lab coat?), what you would do every day (are you a stylist helping someone clean out her closet?), what you would say if you were already this person (are you a world traveler speaking French or a feminist activist discussing the #metoo movement?). Make this person come to life in your mind.

Do one thing. Get up every morning and do one small thing toward living the new identity. Ask yourself how this person would approach their day.

If you're a doctor, you'd get up early, have an invigorating workout, and drink some green juice. If you're a writer, you'd have time blocked off on your calendar to write and would set your alarm to get up early and do it. If you're a world traveler, you'd be reading up on a country you want to visit or cooking meals unique to that country. If you're a spiritual guide to your children, you'd spend time fully engaged with them to ask them what they want to be and help them set a goal to achieve it.

Doing one small thing helps you establish the identity as something very real and gives you the feeling of possibility that you can make it happen. It doesn't matter how small it is — just do one thing every single day.

Change your posture. Change how you carry yourself. Walk taller. Don't suck it in. Don't try to cover yourself up. Look people in the eye. Talk louder. Feel powerful.

It will surprise you to realize how much and how often you shrink and silence yourself once you start doing this. And changing your posture to feel more confident, energized, and powerful really makes you do things differently. Carrying yourself in a powerful way helps you see yourself in a new way, and it's how people with a strong identity express their inner power.

It may feel silly to do these things, but it's not. What's silly — heartbreaking, actually — is how little you expect of yourself and how much you've extinguished the roaring fire that's inside of you to the point that it's barely a flame.

No one has to know what you're doing. And the more impossible or crazy it seems to become the person you're imagining, the more you know you're on the right track.

Thinking of yourself in a bigger way gives you a feeling of possibility, which your subconscious mind will push you to back up with action. The more action you take, the more powerful you feel, and then losing weight will all of a sudden stop being the dominating thought in your mind.

Remember this: you're not doing to get, you're feeling to become.

Your thoughts are behind everything you do, even if you don't notice them — and it's almost certain you don't. And if you're trying to make changes but you're still stuck with the same old, tired thoughts, it's going to be like climbing Mt. Everest.

But it's easy to change them, and now you have a step-by-step process to do it. And if you do the work of writing it all down, you'll get there a whole lot faster. So, commit to doing these exercises, get out that journal, and start right now!

Now let's look at the second half of getting results: changing your habits. Changing your thoughts makes it easier to change your habits, and vice versa. And by doing both simultaneously, you'll get exponential results.

Changing Your Habits

Change might not be fast and it isn't always easy, but with time and effort, almost any habit can be reshaped.

— Charles Duhigg

You just learned how to identify the negative, self-defeating thoughts that hold you back and deliberately and methodically change them. So now it's time to address the actions that you keep taking over and over again that are caused by those thoughts — in other words, your habits.

First, what is a "habit"? Webster's dictionary says that a habit is "an acquired mode of behavior that has become nearly or completely involuntary."

If a habit is involuntary, that means it's not you at work — it's your brain. So, if you're not able to just wake up and change all your habits, you're not a failure. Your brain has put you on autopilot. You've trained it to make you engage automatically in certain behaviors. That's how they became habits.

In his book *The Power of Habit*, Charles Duhigg explores how the brain forms habits. Based on what he learned through his interviews with scientists who research this complex process, he explains that the brain constantly processes information it receives in an effort to become more efficient. It attempts to recognize patterns so that it can save its energy to do more important things, like solve problems.

Once your brain senses a pattern, it rewires itself to take that same action automatically, so it doesn't have to keep remembering to do it. This is how a habit is formed.

This is really important to understand, because all too often, we make judgments about who we are when we're unable to make overnight changes. But it's not about who you are — it's about how you've wired yourself. Habit formation starts in the brain. You don't overeat because you're a loser and can't control yourself. Your brain simply recognized overeating as a pattern so it didn't have to "think" about it anymore.

For you, the pattern became ingrained when you started using food to make yourself feel better — to relieve stress, to shove down painful feelings, to feel less alone. So, your eating habits became established long ago, and because you've spent years entrenching them, they can't be changed overnight, just because you decided to change them.

One of the first distinctions I want you to make is that habits really aren't "good" or "bad" — they just lead to certain outcomes. I don't think anyone would say that binge eating is a good thing, but if you want to change this habit, you have to leave your judgment out of it. The outcome of binge eating is excess weight — and weight isn't "bad," it just is.

Part of changing your habits is taking the shame out of the equation, because as long as you're shaming yourself, you can't solve problems. You want to look at everything you do objectively and see it logically — that way, you can come up with solutions and put them into action.

So, start here: you have habits for a scientific reason, not a moral one. You are not a bad person. You're just a person who has certain habits — and those can be changed.

124

The goal

What usually happens when we try to change our bad habits is that we don't really change them — we just try to get rid of them. We try to completely erase a bad habit and replace it with a good one.

For example, say you want to quit your habit of snacking in the afternoon. What usually happens is that you try to quit doing it cold turkey. So, you commit to not eating anything between the time your kids get home from school and dinner. You're successful the first few days, but then you run out of willpower. You eat a few Girl Scout cookies ("I'll just have a few"), then you shove down some of your kids' Doritos, then you have some string cheese . . . you get the picture.

Then you feel completely out of control, you tell yourself what a loser you are, and the voice in your head says, "Why can't I just stop eating?"
So you give up, quit, and decide that you'll never be able to quit snacking all afternoon because you don't have enough willpower to stop doing it.

This approach places you directly in restrict/binge mode, which of course dieting reinforces because dieting has nothing to do with changing your habits. Dieting means you magically get rid of all your bad habits overnight and do everything completely differently. Then you fail — and binge.

And by the way, it's no wonder that we all fall into this trap of trying to eliminate all our bad habits and replacing them with good ones — we've all been conditioned to do this after dieting for so long.

What you want to do instead is slowly modify a bad habit until it turns into a good habit.

This requires no willpower, so you don't create the resistance involved in trying "not to" that pushes you to binge. Making tiny changes is easy and you get small wins every time you succeed, and these wins keep you motivated and give you momentum. It helps you change your thoughts as you make each small change, which reinforces the changes and makes them stick. And it eliminates that negative voice in your head that shames you for failing.

Trying to ditch a bad habit requires willpower, which creates massive resistance, and when your willpower runs out, you binge and shame yourself. And you do it over and over again, chipping away at your confidence each time.

Let's look at the same scenario but with the small-changes approach instead. Instead of trying not to snack at all, you could allow yourself to snack but change what you snack on. And instead of going straight from Girl Scout cookies to carrot sticks, you could have chocolate-covered raisins. Proactively making this one small change makes you feel confident and in control. Successfully making a better choice motivates you to make another one, and another and another. After an afternoon of making this kind of progress, you're more likely to eat slowly at dinner and not clean your plate.

And as you're making these small changes, your thoughts will naturally start to change — and you'll also be actively identifying them and deliberately changing them, too.

You'll notice that you feel better eating something healthier, and you'll be asking yourself whether the cookies are really that satisfying. You'll think about where the urge to grab them is coming from. You'll be thinking about ways to manage your stress when your kids get home from school if that's the culprit.

You may even decide that you'd rather have the cookies after all. But you may decide to take a few of the cookies outside on your porch — rather than standing at the kitchen counter with the entire box — and slowly eat them while focusing on your thoughts. Or you could set a timer for three minutes when the urge to binge strikes and decide if you really want them when the time's up. (And use that time to write down your thoughts.)

There are hundreds of changes you could make for each habit you want to change, which means that you have hundreds of ways to be successful — as opposed to only one.

This process doesn't take very long, by the way, because of the momentum you get while pairing the small changes with changing how you think. One reinforces the other, and vice versa. And once you master one habit and then add another and another, you start getting exponential success.

Pretty soon, this particular habit of snacking all afternoon starts to become unappealing. And eventually you won't have to try to force yourself not to engage in your bad habits — you'll completely lose interest in them.

Engage in the habit

Part of what makes it hard to change a habit is that people typically go from engagement straight into shame. They try not to binge on chips and then feel like a total failure afterward when they do.

This keeps you stuck, because it prevents you from stepping back from the habit and figuring out what's really going on. It prevents you from seeing the multitude of options available to you to make changes. It prevents you from making a plan to solve the problem — and if you can't problem-solve you can't make progress.

The first step in changing a habit is identifying its associated thoughts — but you can't identify them if you're trying to avoid the habit altogether and then shaming yourself when you give in.

You have to allow yourself to engage in the habit without beating yourself up and investigate what thoughts are causing it. This takes the bullhorn away from your inner critic, because just making the decision to figure out what's happening — before you even make one change — makes you feel confident. You're taking control and proactively doing something, and you give your inner critic nothing to work with.

The main reason this shaming voice arises is because you're trying so hard not to engage in the habit in the first place. You're waking up in the morning and making a promise to yourself that you're not going to mindlessly shove down cookies after lunch. But behind this decision is tremendous fear — fear that you won't be strong enough to stick to your plan when the time comes around. This kind of fear and powerlessness decreases your chances of being successful, and it generates all kinds of resistance, which works against you.

What you want to do is allow yourself to engage. You want to take all the resistance and fear out of it. You don't want to try "not to." Engage fully.

By engaging in the habit, you get to examine the thoughts that are pushing you to engage in it. If it's stress, if it's boredom, if it's because you're telling yourself how much you "love" Doritos — you have to figure out what's going on. You can't identify the thoughts associated with the habit if you're constantly trying to go from A to Z without seeing what's getting you from A to B.

When you engage fully in the habit, you have zero pressure and get right into problem-solving mode. There's no pressure, and there's no evil voice ready to tell you what a loser you are for having the habit, that you're out of control, that you just can't stop eating, blah, blah, blah.

It's such an amazing feeling to just allow yourself to feel peaceful and confident, knowing that you're taking action for a change, rather than being reactive.

This is exactly how all this that you're reading here came about, by the way. I made one decision to just quit inflicting all this pain on myself — to get rid of all the pressure and the noise and the shame and just see what happened.

Once I allowed myself to fully engage in all of my habits and be nice to myself, I was able to see what was really going on — and that I wasn't a lazy, out-of-control loser who just couldn't stop eating. It was like kicking over an ant hill and seeing all the activity going on under the surface. Then all of a sudden, I had a million ways I could make changes and convert my bad habits into something better.

So, step one is to engage fully in your habits — without judging yourself and feeling ashamed.

Choose your own changes

One of the most critical aspects of losing weight permanently by changing your habits is determining which changes you will make. It has less to do with the habits themselves and more on how you *choose* to change them.

As you now know, there's no one-size-fits-all set of instructions that works for everyone, which is basically all a diet is. You have to figure out what works for you and your life: your preferences, your schedule, what your grocery store sells, whether you're 30 or 60, whether you have a family or not.

By determining which changes you will make, you're more likely to be successful, because you'll pick changes that are easy for you to make and then you'll get small wins that keep you motivated to keep going.

But most of all, choosing which changes you'll make means you're taking responsibility and control. One of the biggest reasons dieting doesn't work is because you're allowing someone to tell you what to do rather than doing it yourself. It makes you feel helpless to put someone else in charge or to search for a solution outside yourself.

I've met with so many clients and explained my philosophy and approach and patiently explained that it's more about the way you eat than it is what you're eating. I've explained how if you keep manipulating the foods you eat without changing your thoughts and habits, you'll stay stuck forever in a dieting downward spiral.

And even though they understand what I'm saying and wholeheartedly agree, more often than not the conversation circles back to some version of "Tell me what to eat."

I totally get this. The allure of the magic pill is strong and so, therefore, is the idea that if you take these exact steps, the weight will disappear and your whole life will be transformed overnight.

But that just isn't the way it works. If it did, I wouldn't be writing this book because I would have found the perfect diet that worked for me and for you and for every other woman in the world who's so desperate to lose weight. And we would have all lost it by now and moved on with our lives.

The reason it doesn't work is because there isn't one perfect plan. And even if there was and you followed the magical instructions to the letter, what happens when it's over? You go right back to doing what you've always done, and the weight comes back. No, you have to take control and formulate your own plan — one that will work for you and only you.

Choosing your changes means you're taking responsibility and owning where you are in your life. Taking control means that you're saying, "I can do this." Excuses and desperation go out the window. When you accept responsibility, there's no one to tell you what to do or how to do it. It's a scary but also liberating feeling to know that it's all up to you — scary because now there's no one or nothing to blame but liberating because it feels powerful to take control.

When you take control like this, you'll quickly see that there's no win or lose — there's only a problem to be solved. And there are multiple ways to solve it, and you're capable of figuring out what they are. If you try something that doesn't work, you move on to the next change and try that. And you keep trying and tweaking what you're doing until you figure out what does work.

This is how you really get lasting results, by the way, because the trial-and-error process is how you learn. If you don't learn anything, your results will be short-term.

You learn through trying and failing, and you learn by investigating. Part of figuring out what works is seeking out information to back up what you're doing. You'll be motivated to do things like read up on nutrition and ways to live a healthier life, and this knowledge will help you think differently and reinforces your commitment to changing your life.

Figuring out what you're going to do and what you're going to change is active, not passive. And you're much more likely to be successful when you're taking charge and making your own decisions rather than feeling like you'll never be able to lose weight and that you'll always just be someone who's forever on a diet. And then waste your life being that person.

Add, don't subtract

One of the most effective strategies in making changes to your habits is to add rather than subtract. What I mean by this is to add something healthy to the habit rather than try to take something away.

For example, if you want to stop eating fries when you go out to eat, it's a lot easier to stick with your same order (fries and all) and add a salad to the meal. That way you fill up on something healthy before your main meal comes and are less hungry, which means you'll eat fewer fries.

Contrast this with promising yourself all morning that you're going to be "good" at lunch and not order fries with your meal, hoping you'll have enough willpower to do it, and then caving in and scarfing the whole plate down.

Or look at this example from my life. When I was in college, I used to eat at least once a week at a restaurant that had blackened chicken pasta on the menu. I went there with my girlfriends, and we drank wine and talked and laughed. I loved this dish so much that it was the only thing I ever ordered.

I knew it was unhealthy — I was always stuffed to the point of feeling sick after I ate it, and it was so spicy it kept me awake. I tried on several occasions to order a salad instead, but as soon as I sat down, I knew I was going to order my favorite meal. And my inability to make a different choice made me feel like a failure.

But one night, I asked the waiter if I could add broccoli to the meal. This simple, positive act made me feel good about myself and like I had done something healthy — even though I still ate the whole dish.

This one small addition to my unhealthy meal led to more changes. I started asking for tomato sauce instead of cream sauce. I started asking for the chicken to be grilled instead of blackened. I started adding more vegetables, which eventually became substitutes for the chicken. Ultimately, the dish became a whole new meal.

The really exciting thing about these changes was that it made me see the whole experience differently. I realized that it wasn't just the meal that was the problem: I was eating too much, and I was also drinking too much and eating too late.

Making these distinctions (in other words, changing my thoughts) made it even easier to make more healthy changes — at this restaurant and at all the others where I ate. And it all started with one simple addition. (In fact, I no longer eat meat, and I cannot imagine a time when I actually enjoyed a full plate of blackened chicken, swimming in cream sauce.)

Adding something to what you're already doing is far, far easier than trying to eliminate something — particularly if it's an entire habit. And because it's so easy to accomplish, you get a small win that keeps you moving forward.

And while you're getting that small win by making a simple healthy addition, you're making distinctions that you can use to make better decisions the next time. You disrupt your pattern, which makes you think differently and question your assumptions. For example, how delicious is it actually to eat an enormous plate of pasta that could easily be a meal for three people? And is it truly satisfying to shove down a meal so spicy that it keeps you awake all night?

Once you start thinking differently and questioning the thoughts that are going on in your mind, you can easily see that what you're telling yourself isn't necessarily true, which makes it a lot easier to change the habit.

Your goal is to gradually modify a bad habit until becomes a good habit, and making small additions to what you're already doing makes this happen automatically. Your healthy additions will crowd out all the things that makes this habit bad, and then it will slowly start to resemble a good habit.

And because adding them one by one is easy to do, the more small wins you get and the more confidence you build. And the more confident you feel, the easier it is to keep making changes.

Tiny tweaks and small wins

After years of dieting and failing, over and over again, I cannot overstate the importance of building confidence.

One of the biggest reasons you stay stuck in the dieting cycle is a feeling of being powerless to change anything. You stay stuck because of the belief that it will never happen because you're out of control around food or that you don't have enough willpower to stick to a diet. You stay stuck because you feel stuck — and you feel stuck because you don't feel capable of changing anything.

Having confidence is a key element of being able to make changes, because to even decide that you will make a change requires confidence. Then it requires more confidence to push through the trial-and-error process that comes with figuring out something on your own, because you will most definitely "fail" from time to time on your journey of solving the problem. And when there's no road map and no one else telling you what to do, you have to believe in yourself.

So where do you get this confidence? You develop it, slowly and methodically, by getting small wins. You get these wins by making microchanges that make you instantly successful and boost your confidence.

With every small win, you move away from the person who feels desperate and powerless and become someone who's powerful and in control. Feeling capable and confident is the fuel for this whole process — changing your thoughts and habits is what's on the surface, but the power to make those changes is coming from belief in yourself that you have what it takes to make those changes. And the more of them you make, the more confident you feel.

Think about small wins and building confidence this way. It's like running a marathon. Not only is a marathon composed of 26 one-mile runs, which you have to complete to cross the finish line, you also become more capable of crossing that finish line because of the endurance you build with every one of those smaller runs. And every one-mile small win increases your confidence that you have what it takes to go all the way.

You don't wake up, roll out of bed, and run a marathon. That's dieting mentality. You wake up, roll out of bed, and do one small thing after another — and those small wins add up to your own personal, weight-loss medal.

134

Small wins are the key to everything. And the way to begin is to make sure that you get one right out of the gate. This is especially true at the beginning when your confidence is low. You want to set yourself up for success, so that means creating a plan that gives you multiple small wins immediately. This is why choosing your own changes is critical, because only you know which actions will be easy for you to take and which ones will be harder.

You'll come up with a list of possible changes, and you'll start with the easiest ones to ensure that you get immediate small wins. Then — and this is critical — if one of the changes you pick isn't working so well, you change course and pick another one. You'll have plenty of options to choose from, which means there's no failure.

The final key element of this process is that small wins add up over time, and they compound. You start becoming exponentially successful and seeing results with every change you make. To use our marathon analogy, the closer you get to the finish line, the faster you cross it.

This is one of the most beautiful parts of the whole habit/thought change process. The more thoughts and habits you deliberately change, the more your thoughts and habits start to change automatically.

And all of a sudden, you start becoming this new person who wants to do healthy things instead of having to force herself to do them. You start seeking out information on your own and finding new opportunities to do things that make you healthier and stronger. And pretty soon your previous thoughts and habits seem foreign, as though they belong to another person — and that's because you're no longer that person.

At first it won't seem like anything major is happening. Especially after being so conditioned to do everything all-or-nothing and feeling desperate for immediate results. But be patient. You'll spend a certain amount of time climbing the base of your mountain — but pretty soon it will be a sprint to the summit.

How to do it

Remember your two main goals: 1) challenge and change your thoughts and 2) gradually modify a bad habit until it becomes a good habit.

Here's the step-by-step process for changing your habits:

1. Get out your journal and brainstorm the top 3 to 5 habits that you want to change. Write them down.

2. Order them from easiest to change to hardest to change.

3. Start with the easiest habit and write down every single microchange you could make to that habit to transform it into a good habit (use the list of 45 tweaks at the end of this chapter for ideas).

For example, if you want to stop bingeing on cookies, you could portion out the number of cookies you'll eat, you could eat them outside instead of in front of the computer, you could switch from Chips Ahoy to a healthier organic cookie, or you could eat a handful of blueberries or run up and down the stairs three times before you eat them.

When you're coming up with changes, don't use elimination strategies at first; start with additions rather than subtractions until you gain confidence.

4. Pick the 5 to 7 strategies that would be the easiest for you to implement.

5. Choose the first 2 or 3 to work on this week.

6. On day 1, engage fully in the habit and write down your thoughts: what leads up to the habit, what you think about while you engage in the habit, and what you think about after you engage in it.

7. On day 2, start adding your tiny tweaks. Add the first one and master it. If you have trouble, don't worry, pick another one. Small

wins are what you're after. Your goal is to master at least two per week. If they're super easy and you feel inspired to add another one, go ahead — but don't overload yourself. Take it as slow as you need to.

8. Continue with your thought-changing as you add the tweaks. Write down every single thought and feeling you have. You'll be tempted to slack off, but please don't! Writing it down is critical to your success. You'll always be surprised at what shows up on the page, and it makes altering your habits much easier and way more effective.

9. Once your first habit starts to change, start on the second one.

10. Continue modifying the first habit while you work on the second one. Continue implementing more tweaks from your list and changing the thoughts associated with the first habit and the new distinctions you're making.

11. Reward yourself every time you change one of your habits. Go get a pedicure, buy a new outfit, have dinner with a girlfriend, sleep in one morning. Having a reward to work toward is incredibly motivating — and you deserve to feel good after all the misery you've subjected yourself to!

Whatever change you successfully make is a win, no matter how small it is. And there is no failure — there's only learning what works and what doesn't. It's a lifetime process, really, and the more you start shifting your perspective, the easier it will get. You're no longer going to fall into the trap of going balls-to-the wall to get results that don't last — now you're committed to making long-term changes that actually stick.

The more changes you make, the more momentum you get, and the more confident you become. Pretty soon, your good habits will start to crowd the bad ones out, and your life will look totally different. And you will *be* totally different!

Strategies for improving habits

Here are a few overall strategies to consider while you're making these changes that will make it easier to change your habits.

Make the bad habit painful

Think about some of the good habits you have right now. There are definitely several that are super easy for you to engage in, and you don't have to force yourself to do them. To put it another way, you associate more pain with not doing them than you do with doing them. You've developed positive associations with these habits, so they're effortless.

For example, I'm an extreme morning person. I've trained myself to wake up early for so long that I don't even need an alarm anymore. I don't have to set an alarm and hit snooze ten times, just to drag myself out of bed, hating every second of it.

The reason why is that it would be far more painful for me to sleep in. If I sleep in, I miss the time of enjoying a solo cup of coffee, reading something inspiring, writing down my goals, and planning out my day. If I sleep in, I won't feel like my best self when I wake my kids up for school — I'd be a lot more impatient and frazzled if I didn't get up and have that time. (This isn't to say that I never sleep in, because I do. But even when I do, my body clock still goes off at 4:00 am.)

The key is that I developed this habit over time. I used to sleep until noon in college, and I cannot even imagine doing this now. But I had to suffer the consequences of sleeping in all the time to figure out that my day went a whole lot better if I got up early. I learned over time to associate sleeping in with pain and to associate getting up early with pleasure. (The pleasure/pain concept is one of Tony Robbins's core teachings if you want to read more about this.)

To look at it another way, the pleasure I got from sleeping late wasn't enough to outweigh the pain it caused, and the pain of waking up early was insignificant in comparison to the pleasure I got from doing it. However, to figure all this out, I had to start waking up early — I had to engage in the activity to weigh its pros and cons.

So, a very useful tactic is to think of a good habit you have and figure out how you associate pleasure with doing it, and how not doing it would cause you pain. Think about how you developed this habit and how you learned to associate it with pleasure.

Are you a neat freak? Then you associate pain with being disorganized. You derive pleasure in keeping things orderly, and the pain it would cause you to live in disarray makes this habit easy for you. But for someone who finds chaos a pleasurable state, having to weed out closets and drawers is about the worst thing ever. They associate pleasure with going with the flow and think that having a squared-off, military-like existence is painful. (I find it delightful, however.)

Are you always punctual? Then you associate more pain with being late than you do with the pleasure of not having to show up on time. You associate being on time with pleasure and being late with pain. But people who are chronically late think of being on time as being a slave to the clock and find pleasure in not having to commit to anyone.

So, think about a bad habit you have and want to change. Think about how you're currently associating pleasure with it and how you could instead start associating it with pain. Think of the negative consequences of that habit and question whether the "pleasure" you think you're getting is actually pleasurable.

Part of the reason it feels hard to change a habit is that you're attaching so much pleasure to it. But if you look closely, there are powerful painful consequences to engaging in it — you're just not focusing on them.

Give yourself a break

The process of changing your thoughts and habits requires work — and if you don't consistently put in the work, nothing is going to change. However, it's also important to give yourself breaks.

There's no time limit to this process — you're in it for the long haul. You definitely don't want to overwhelm yourself by trying to change too much at once, but if you find that you've bitten off more than you can chew, it's okay to pull back and slow down.

The key to being successful at anything in life is choosing a mindset that supports you. The dieting mindset you're used to is the polar opposite of what you need to have. Going all or nothing, running out of willpower, failing, and quitting will get you nowhere and will keep you stuck. You have to choose the mindset of getting a little bit better, every single day. And to do this you have to support yourself.

And because life circumstances change, your mindset has to change with them. Some days you need to push yourself harder, and others you need to take a break and relax. The key is balance, and only you know which mindset to choose.

So, if you feel overloaded, take a break. And if you slip up, definitely give yourself a mental and emotional break.

Give yourself an out

This is a psychological trick that works extremely well. It's counterintuitive, but it works. If there's a habit I'm working on changing, I give myself the option of doing it, even as I'm trying to stop doing it. In other words, I give myself an out.

Here's how it works: if you give yourself the option of doing whatever it is you're trying not to do, you actually increase your odds of successfully not doing it. That's because you take all the pressure off yourself, and you decrease the resistance that wrecks everything.

For example, say you're going to dinner with some friends, and your goal is to stop eating fries with your meal. Say you've got your plan in place to add a side salad to your meal to fill up on first, in an effort to eat fewer fries. You feel motivated because of having this easy change in your back pocket that will surely give you a small win.

To increase the effectiveness of your plan, tell yourself that you can have all the fries you want. This takes every single bit of pressure off you and eliminates the stress you're so used to feeling when it comes to food and eating — the fear-based mentality of food being your adversary and you being powerless over it.

The interesting thing is that when you give yourself the option of doing whatever it is you're trying not to do, you rarely take it. That's because you're putting yourself in control of the situation rather than feeling out of control when you encounter it.

Give yourself an out, particularly if what you're trying not to do is especially challenging. And even if you do "fail" and indulge in your out, you won't feel as bad about it since you gave yourself permission.

Show up

I have a saying that runs through my head every single morning, as soon as I wake up. Here it is: *Get up, show up, do the work.*

This saying is like gold, especially if I'm not feeling very motivated. That's because it helps me ignore the voice in my head that tells me how long it's going to take me to do something or how painful it's going to be. It helps me steer clear of all those mental weeds and walk directly to the actions I need to take to accomplish something.

Even better, it firmly cements this fact into my brain: all I have to do, literally, is show up. I don't have to have it all figured out and I don't have to do it perfectly. All I know is that if I just show up, things will happen.

Showing up works well for just about anything. If I need to work out but dread doing it, all I have to do is get on the treadmill and the run happens automatically. If I need to write something but feel like I have nothing to say, all I have to do is open the laptop and the words come out. If I want to eat a healthy lunch but don't feel like making one, all I have to do is get out the veggies and the lunch gets made.

This trick is especially helpful if you've slipped up and are feeling bad about yourself. You don't have to wallow in self-pity or feel disappointed, and you don't have to wreck all the good progress you can make today. All you have to do is get up, show up, and get back to work.

Sometimes we feel so far away from a goal that it feels like little steps don't make a dent. And this is when discouragement sets in — and with it, inaction. But just keep in mind that all you have to do is show up, and you'll stay on track. And before you know it, your goal is achieved.

Get back to the basics

I have five habits that have nothing to do with food or eating that make me feel healthy and in control. And no matter what happened yesterday, I know I can wake up and do these five things to get myself back on track. They instantly give me the "it's a brand new day" feeling I need to keep going, especially if I've slipped up.

1. Sweat. Tell yourself all you need to do is break a sweat. You don't need to have an hour-long, hard-core workout session. Just break a sweat. Sweating makes you feel like you're getting things moving and the clean-out process started. And taking a steam or a sauna counts!

2. Hydrate. There's nothing easier than drinking water to make you feel like you're doing something healthy. Put bottles by your bedside table, in your bathroom, in your car, next to your computer, or anywhere you spend time. Drinking water couldn't be easier, and not only do you instantly feel like you're making progress, you're getting closer to your weight-loss goal by staying hydrated.

3. Exfoliate. This is one of my favorites. Scrubbing off all the dead skin makes you feel like a new person, and it's super relaxing. You don't need anything fancy — sugar and olive oil is perfect. Doing something like this is part of the self-care that's required in living a healthy life, and giving yourself a mini spa treatment is well-deserved after working as hard as you no doubt do.

4. Nap. Ok, this one is hard for people to accept, because we've all been so conditioned to feel lazy if we do. But if you feel tired, please promise me you will take a nap — even if it's just for fifteen minutes. And feel good about it!

Don't treat yourself like a drill sergeant and push yourself until you collapse, because that's a good way to make sure you binge on something. Taking a break and resting for a little while is way healthier than shoving down some potato chips because you've pushed yourself past the point.

5. De-stress. Feeling constantly stressed keeps cortisol flowing through your veins, which makes you more likely to binge eat and store fat. Make a list of three or four easy things you can do to relax when you feel overwhelmed, irritated, or stressed.

Light a candle, listen to classical music, go sit outside. Doing things like this not only helps you calm down, but it also helps you feel more loving toward yourself and therefore less resistant of your body.

6. Bonus tip: Don't hit the bottle. Don't hit it so hard, anyway. Unless you have a problem with alcohol and truly need to quit, take this tip to heart and decrease the amount of alcohol you consume.

Drinking alcohol doesn't just make you forget your problems, but it also makes you forget about your goals and your commitment to them. You're more likely to backslide into your old habits when you drink, and you're also more likely to give yourself license to binge and overdo it, especially if you're an emotional eater.

Take a day off once in a while, intersperse water with your drinks, or do something on your de-stress list to relax instead. You deserve better than to wreck all your progress by getting hammered at girls' night out. And you definitely don't need a hangover to deal with the next day. You will feel so much better and more in control by choosing to decrease your alcohol intake, I promise you. It's just not worth it.

Try these strategies out as you change your thoughts and habits. They really helped me speed up my progress and hit my weight-loss goal faster, and they also help keep me on track as I continue my commitment to living the healthiest life I possibly can.

Now let's look at some habits that are useful to get rid of. Some of them may not be so obvious, and they're likely hindering your progress without you being aware of it.

45 Habit Tweaks

Change How You Eat

Sit somewhere different
Eat at a table (no screens)
Add fresh herbs to your meal
Add a piece of fruit to your meal
Play relaxing music while you eat
Leave the last bite of food on your plate
Put your fork down between bites
Set a timer while you eat
Order half of your food to go
Eat a mint halfway through your meal
Drink a glass of water before you eat
Drink a glass of water at the first sign of hunger
Order a healthier dessert (don't eliminate it)
Substitute a salad for fries
Add lemon/lime to your water
Breathe deeply for one minute before eating
Eat a piece of fruit before you eat your meal

Change What You Do

Plant fresh herbs in your kitchen
Cook at least one meal a day
Play relaxing music while you cook
Cut up veggies to put in the fridge
Dress up before you eat (don't slouch around)
Use your good china or crystal
Prep your next meal after you finish the first one (so you don't
just grab whatever)

Buy a new cookbook
Buy a new kitchen gadget (like a spiralizer or a mini chop)
Call a friend when the urge to binge strikes

Change How You Move

Set out your workout clothes the night before
Sign up for a new workout class
Ease into your workout with a baby step (get on the treadmill and see what happens)
Get a rebounder and bounce 10 minutes a day
Walk with light weights
Recruit a friend to exercise with you
Buy a new workout outfit
Set your alarm 10 minutes early to stretch
Sign up for an active event (like a 5K)
Pace while you talk on the phone
Park farther away in the parking lot
Exercise between tasks while you clean your house (do lunges or push-ups)
Stretch while you watch television
Take a break at work and walk a flight of stairs
Walk the mall/airport concourse
Take a cooking class
Give yourself a non-food reward
Try a new restaurant

Small, incremental changes are the key
to staggering long-term results.

Habits to Break

A bad habit never disappears miraculously.
It's an undo-it-yourself project.

— *Abigail van Buren*

I generally don't like speaking in negatives — I prefer to phrase everything in the positive. But if any of these habits are familiar to you, you would be doing yourself a favor to eliminate them.

As always, your goal is to gradually modify bad habits until they become good habits, but so I can spare you the repetition and make my point more easily, I'm going to talk about habits you should break.

Mindless eating

Mindless eating is basically exactly what it sounds like: eating without thinking. It's eating without being fully present during the act of eating.

Eating mindlessly is very familiar to those of us who eat emotionally, because emotional eating is what's behind eating this way. You eat mindlessly because the act of eating is what's filling you up — not the food that you're eating.

I fully relate to eating like this. It took me years to stop sitting down in front of the television or my computer to eat. I had trained myself to take a break from all the stress, sit down with whatever it was I was eating, and zone out while I was eating it.

The problem with doing this is that you can't notice the feeling of fullness that tells you when to quit. Actually, when you're zoned out like this, you don't notice much of anything. But that's the whole point. What you're looking for is the temporary escape, the check-out.

The problem is that eating mindlessly reinforces you using food as a reward, and it also makes you eat more than you need, which equals weight gain.

It feels hard to stop doing this if you've trained yourself to check out this way. But it is possible. If I can do it, anyone can!

Strategies

Make a conscious decision. When you feel the impulse to grab something and zone out, stop, take a breath, and decide what you're going to do. It's okay to eat something, but choose what it's going to be — do it consciously. Even if it's a bag of M&Ms, be deliberate about it. Then decide where you're going to sit and how long you're going to sit there. Just being present while you make the choice — even if it's not the perfect choice — is a step in the right direction.

Get away from the screen. Sitting in front of your laptop or the television is the most effective way to make sure you zone out and eliminate every shred of consciousness. Take the food you've decided to eat and go somewhere where you can focus, outside, if possible. Being in nature helps you slow down and connect with the experience of eating. If you can't go outside, sit down in a quiet room (even if you have to lock yourself in your bedroom and hide from your kids) and consciously eat.

Do prep work. Set aside 10 to 15 minutes of non-negotiable prep time each day to make healthy snacks and prep for meals. Preparing what you're going to eat in advance really helps you stop grabbing whatever's sitting around, and planning and prepping means you're automatically present and conscious so you're already in the right frame of mind when you eat. You're also more likely to eat whatever it is you took the time to prepare, so you'll eat healthier.

Hold off. If you eat mindlessly at the beginning of the day, you're more likely to continue doing it the rest of the day because you've opened the floodgates. I call this "feeding the beast."

If you feel the urge to do your zone-out, stop and wait a few minutes — then make your decision. If you can prevent yourself from eating mindlessly at the outset of your day, you're more likely to continue resisting the urge as the day goes on. You get small wins every time you stop yourself altogether or even if you choose to eat but do it consciously.

Rewarding yourself with food

Rewarding yourself with food is similar to mindless eating because eating mindlessly is a kind of reward. Using food as a reward does nothing but keep you stuck, fluctuating eternally at around the same weight and having to endure the back-and-forth in your head going on and on about how good you were and you deserve to blow it out or how good you're going to be today after yesterday's binge.

You're preventing yourself from having a normal relationship with food by setting up this punishment/reward cycle. You restrict yourself from eating, then reward yourself for not eating. Then you feel bad about the reward you gave yourself, so you punish yourself the next day by not eating — then reward yourself again.

Food isn't a reward — it's something to enjoy. And you can't ever truly enjoy your food if you're using it this way.

Strategies

Stop doing "checks and balances." Thinking long-term is generally a good thing, but sometimes you need to think short-term — specifically, the current moment. Focus only on what you're eating right now. Don't think about cutting calories at this meal so you can binge at the next meal. Don't think about all the healthy choices you made earlier, so you can level it out with the binge you "deserve" to have.

Focus on what you're doing in the moment, and make deliberate choices that support your health, one after another. Just keep doing the next right thing, regardless of what happened last week, yesterday, or at lunch.

Find other rewards. Light a candle, go for a walk, call a friend — or even sit in front of the television or computer . . . but without the food. Get out your journal and make a list of things you can do to take the place of mindless eating, and run down your list anytime you feel the urge.

Eating too fast

When you eat too fast, you feel out of control, and this is the polar opposite of what you need to feel if you're going to change your life.

Eating too fast is a byproduct of the first two habits I just talked about. If you eat mindlessly to check out or use food to reward yourself, it's guaranteed you're going to eat too fast and overeat. If you're enjoying and appreciating the food you're eating, you eat consciously and slowly. If you're using food to fill a void, it's the eating that's filling you up — not the food itself.

But if you can learn to slow down while you eat, you'll automatically eliminate the first two habits. If you eat slowly and deliberately, it pulls you directly into the moment so you're no longer shoving it down mindlessly. And if you eat with an appreciation of the food and how it's fueling your body, it stops being a reward and becomes what it should be: a way to nourish and care for yourself.

Eating slowly also helps you feel in control, which decreases the urge to binge. It helps you think more clearly, so you make better decisions about what to eat. It helps you pay attention to what you're thinking and helps you identify the feeling of fullness you miss when you binge eat. And it helps you see that you're able to be satisfied with less food.

Finally, if you eat slowly, you can eat just about anything you want!

Strategies

- Prepare your food slowly and deliberately
- Put your fork down between bites
- Take smaller bites
- Play relaxing music while you eat
- Breathe and be in the moment
- Set a timer for 20 minutes and use the entire time to eat
- Drink a full bottle of water during your meal

Never cooking

If you want to lose weight, you have to have a healthy relationship with food. And if you want to have a healthy relationship with food, you have to connect with it. And if you're going to connect with your food, you have to prepare it — which means you have to cook it.

Eating food out of a package, eating fast food, and even eating meals that are delivered to your door all disconnect you in some way from the food you eat. Being disconnected from your food fuels your unhealthy relationship with it, which results in weight gain, which keeps you stuck in the dieting cycle.

One of the most effective and things I ever did to help me escape an unhealthy relationship with food was to teach myself how to cook. To be clear, I'm no chef, and I don't have one of those fancy kitchens with stainless-steel appliances and a pantry full of exotic ingredients. I don't have amazing technique, and I'm pretty sure if Gordon Ramsey saw me cook, he would kick me out of Hell's Kitchen.

However, I taught myself to do some basic things that make me feel like a gourmet cook and that have completely changed my relationship with food. My culinary prowess used to be limited to boiling pasta and pouring cheap tomato sauce on it. Now I sauté shallots and garlic with my stir fry, I make fresh pesto sauce (it takes about three minutes and is so much better than store-bought it's ridiculous), and I create my own casseroles. I've even experimented with making sushi, using phyllo dough, and baking macarons. More than a few times what I've made has been disastrous, but that's not what matters. What matters is the effort, because making an effort means you're taking control.

I think we make cooking unnecessarily hard. We assume that we don't know how (how can you if you've never even tried?), that it takes a huge amount of time and effort (it doesn't), and that it's a complete chore (when it's actually creative and fun).

There are so many benefits to cooking. It's healthier, because you use fresh ingredients and you get more variety. It helps you stop bingeing, because when you make it yourself, you're not going to waste all your hard work by mindlessly shoving it down. It helps you branch out and try new foods. It helps you feel creative, which builds your confidence. And it improves your distorted relationship with food, because when you participate in the preparation of it, you're less afraid of it and feel less out of control around it.

Even if you just buy pre-grilled chicken from the deli and thaw some frozen broccoli, that's better than eating a Lean Cuisine. You don't have to go from fast food to five star — take baby steps. And there's no pressure to even become five star. All you have to do is take control, just a little bit, and connect with the food you eat.

Strategies

Make one new meal per week. If you hardly ever cook, commit to making at least one dinner per week. If you cook pretty often, commit to trying one new dish per week, especially if you're in a rut. And if you're an experienced cook and do it regularly — congratulations, you're way ahead of the game! If you're already accomplished, come up with healthier versions of what you already make.

Buy a cookbook. Even if you have several, go out and buy a beautiful new cookbook that inspires you. Take some time during the week to browse through it and look for recipes to try out. Use this time as one of your non-food, self-care rewards. Set the cookbook on the counter to remind yourself of your commitment to taking control and living a healthy life.

Do some meal prep. I'll return to this tactic again and again, because it's so important in your ability to take control. Chop up fruits and vegetables ahead of time to increase your odds of cooking and not grabbing something to heat up in the microwave. Wash some fresh herbs or rinse the vegetables you need to get ready for the healthy dinner you're making.

Get organized. Keep your kitchen clean and organized. You can't take control of food if your kitchen is out of control. You're not going to want to cook anything if you can't stand being in your cluttered kitchen, and you can't stock it with new ingredients if there's no space. I'll dive into this in more detail in the next chapter, but do everything you can to ensure your kitchen is prepped for success.

Engaging in other "binge" behaviors

Extreme behaviors create imbalance, which has to be righted. If you exercise obsessively and push yourself to the limit, you're going to quit working out at all. If you work ten-hour days, you're going to spend your weekends engrossed in a Netflix binge. And if you starve yourself, you're going to eventually cave and eat everything in sight.

The bad news is that if you're an all-or-nothing person like I am, your tendency is to exhibit binge-like behaviors in every aspect of your life. You probably rush around, feeling like you have to get everything done at once, with a to-do list a mile long. You're a workaholic. You're a perfectionist and can't rest until your house looks immaculate. And all of these extreme behaviors mean you're more likely to binge eat. (Trust me, I know.)

When you go all-or-nothing and push yourself excessively hard, you're going to seek out some sort of reward: drinking wine, zoning out in front of the television, or binge eating. Maybe all three.

A simple way to stop binge eating is to slow down in every aspect of your life. When you start moving at a slower pace, it spills over into your eating habits. And when you slow down, your thoughts slow down — then you can more easily spot the ones that are holding you back.

You don't have to stop working hard or doing a good job, just pull it back a little bit and breathe. Take everything more slowly, and don't be so hard on yourself. Enjoy your life more, and you'll be less likely to use food to make yourself feel better.

Strategies

Stop being a workaholic. Even if you don't have a 9-to-5 job, you may still be a workaholic. Unplug your phone for at least one hour a day. Spend that time doing something creative and relaxing, like journaling or cooking. Limit your email checking to twice per day. Use at least one half-day per week doing something that involves self-care (get a manicure, read a book, take a bath). Don't add already-completed tasks to your to-do list just so you can check them off (yes, I do that). You can work hard, but you don't have to be a martyr. The laundry doesn't all have to be done today.

Stop trying to be perfect. This is another habit to quit that I'm going to talk about in more detail: stop putting so much pressure on yourself. All that resistance makes it more likely that you'll binge to make yourself feel better. You don't have to be the perfect mom, employee, wife, or woman. Give yourself a break.

Move slower. As I just said, whatever you're doing, do it more slowly. Walk across the room more slowly, drive more slowly, put the dishes away more slowly. Get in the habit of slowing way, way down. It will help you eat more slowly.

Focusing obsessively on how you look

It's hard not to think about what you look like when you want to lose weight, because part of the reason you have that goal is to change your appearance. But focusing obsessively on your looks creates resistance — both emotional and physical.

It creates emotional resistance because it's demoralizing to think about how horrible you look (or think you look), which amplifies your inner critic, making it worse. And it creates physical resistance, because you start contorting your body into all sorts of unnatural positions to hide the parts you don't like.

Fighting against your own body like this is the ultimate resistance, and it disconnects you from your inner self and all its wisdom and strength, which is what you need most of all if you want to make a transformation happen.

You don't want to waste any more time thinking about what you look like, and you don't want to continue hating your body and feeling disconnected from it. You need to feel whole and complete already, even if you're not totally happy with how you look. This requires self-love and self-acceptance, which don't automatically appear once you start this process. It takes practice to get to there.

It's true that confidence is attractive, and I'm sure you've experienced this in your own life. Have you ever met someone who's physically beautiful by anyone's standards but has no confidence? It makes that person less attractive, meaning literally less *attract*-ive — this person doesn't attract you to them because of their lack of connection with themselves.

Contrast this with someone who isn't traditionally beautiful but who feels confident and is expressing inner beauty. You're attracted to people like this, because they feel comfortable with themselves and connected with themselves. You're not noticing their wrinkles or the extra weight they're carrying around their midsection or how untoned their arms are. All you're feeling is their inner confidence being radiated, and that is powerfully attractive.

So how do you do stop obsessing constantly about what you look like, particularly when your main goal is to lose weight? You have to start focusing more on how you feel than on how you look. The more you get in touch with how you feel, the more you'll naturally gravitate toward more healthy behaviors that make you feel good. When you focus on how you feel, you'll learn to recognize true hunger and consciously respond, and you'll learn to listen to what your body needs.

The good news is that this process of changing your thoughts and habits builds your confidence, one small win at a time, and it helps you focus on living in a healthier way — and the more you do these things, how you look will start to change effortlessly.

Strategies

Throw out your scale. Stop weighing yourself to see how much you've lost or gained. When you constantly weigh yourself, all you're doing is letting an arbitrary measurement determine how you act. If the number is something you like, you tend to take actions consistent with success. But if the number isn't what you wanted to see, you feel bad and want to give up and quit — and therefore take actions that are the exact opposite of what you should do.

Change how you carry yourself. Instead of constricting your body, relax and allow yourself to move more slowly. Walk more slowly, and try to make your movements more deliberate. Feel in control with every move you make. The more relaxed and centered and deliberate you are — mentally and physically — the more confident you feel.

Walk with certainty, stand taller, breathe more deeply. Even if you don't look the way you want to (yet), by carrying yourself this way, you will evolve into the person you imagine yourself being.

Go makeup free for a day. Not to make you feel worse about yourself but to shift your attention. If you're not wearing makeup, there's no need to constantly check yourself in the mirror to see if you need more lipstick or if your mascara is flaking off. The less you do this, the more you can focus on how you feel. You probably miss a lot of great insights and connections with other people because of always worrying about what you look like — I know I sometimes do . . . still!

We've all been conditioned to obsess about what we look like, and it's no wonder. But just take a day to chill out from all that. It's really so liberating. And if it's too crazy to contemplate, just do it at home.

Trying to be perfect

It's no wonder we're all conditioned to strive for perfection, because that's all we see. The media is filled with airbrushed images that create the illusion of perfection. What's important to remember is that it's just that — an illusion. It's not real.

But even though we all know that, we're still deeply affected by it. And we've been so conditioned by it that it narrows our focus to getting instant results instead of seeing ourselves as whole and experiencing our lives as a series of never-ending attempts to becoming who we're capable of being. We all get lost in the fantasy that if we could look perfect, our lives would be perfect.

Striving for perfection, something that doesn't actually exist, will keep you stuck. For one thing, if it doesn't exist, you will never achieve it. And for another, feeling like you're always falling short makes you feel awful and prevents you from taking the actions necessary to actually achieve the goal. If you feel bad about your lack of results, you'll be paralyzed into inaction — into perfection paralysis.

If you constantly stare at your muffin top, you won't do sit-ups. If you focus on how heavy your legs look, you're not going to go for a run. If you're thinking about how fat you look in your yoga pants, you're not going to take an exercise class. You'll want to curl up and eat ice cream. And then you'll never even do the bare minimum required to get close to your goal.

You have to drop the mindset that perfection is what you want. You don't have to be content with mediocre results — but you don't have to keep trying in vain to achieve something that doesn't exist in the first place.

Strategies

Saturate yourself with success. Read success books, seek out information, talk to people who have goals. Stop inundating yourself with airbrushed images and pictures of women who look perfect. Focus on creating something meaningful. Set a big goal for yourself. Doing this will automatically result in the lesser goal of losing weight. And again, the more confident you feel, the better you will look.

Reflect. This is serious business, committing to a healthy life — one that is healthy physically, emotionally, and mentally. It takes time, serious self-reflection and honesty, and effort to do the work necessary to make permanent changes. Feel good that you've decided to do this.

You have to spend time in focused reflection to make all this happen. Getting still, thinking, processing, and writing it all down is a requirement. But the good news is that doing all of this reinforces your belief in yourself and decreases your emotional investment in the fantasy of perfection, where you have the perfect home and you wear the perfect clothes and you have the perfect body.

Strengthening your inner self helps you let go of the Instagram life — where everyone else only appears to have the perfect life.

Be your biggest supporter. Again, the deadliest thing about wanting to be perfect is that it gives your inner critic a bullhorn. The more you fall short, the worse you feel, and the more paralyzed you get.

Resolve to be your own best friend. Talk yourself up. Focus on what you love about yourself. Think of all the ways you excel and every amazing thing you've ever achieved. And, of course, write it all down.

Then remind yourself daily, multiple times per day, of everything praise-worthy about you. Then praise yourself!

Starting over again and again

If you've dieted over and over again for years, you're familiar with constantly starting over. This is epitomized by the "I'll start on Monday" mentality.

You work really hard, you go full force, you run out of willpower, you fail, you give up and quit — and you start all over.

This mindset is fueled by the mistaken belief that you've failed. We're all conditioned to wrongly believe that trying and not achieving a goal equals failure. This simply isn't true, and by believing it you train yourself to quit give up a lot sooner than you should. (Actually, you should never give up.)

The truth is that you're always one step closer to your goal, even if you can't see it. You're always making progress, and that's a fact, because by taking any action you become a different person than you were. If your situation isn't different, *you* are different. You've made a new distinction, however minute, that turns you into more of the person you are capable of being. Even if the action didn't result in the outcome you intended.

In other words, if you fell short of a goal, you made a misstep. But even that is good because it means you learned something. And you can use that knowledge to do it differently next time. There are never failures, only mistakes — and mistakes aren't failures.

Strategies

Shake it up. When you get trapped in the start-over rut, you tend to do the same things over and over again. You take the same actions, thinking you're going to get the same result. Try mixing it up a little. Do a different work out. Try a new dish. Think different thoughts.

You don't need to keep beating your head against the wall and considering yourself a failure when all along it was your approach that may not have been working. Try something new for a change — the energy you generate by doing something different may be all you need to reach the goal.

Course-correct. Make tiny course corrections along the way. Getting into the habit of making tiny adjustments gets you out of the all-or-nothing mindset that keeps you starting over again at square one. There are multiple paths to any destination, but if you keep going back home and repacking your bag after every wrong turn, you'll never get to where you want to go.

Every time you "fail," try to figure out what didn't work (and no, it wasn't you). Make a list of three small changes you could make to modify what you did. You'll slowly start to get results and shake yourself out of the feeling that you have to start all over again.

Create small wins. One of the cornerstones of this whole process! Make it easy for you to get small victories, especially at the beginning. The easier they are, the better. This lines up perfectly with course correction, because making tiny shifts gives you the small wins you need to stay motivated and march along the path to goal achievement.

Commiserating with your friends

It's hard to lose weight the older you get.
It's hard to find time to exercise when you have kids.
We need to blow it out tonight — we've been so good all week!

Does any of this sound familiar? Commiserating with your friends and saying things like this will keep you stuck right where you are, for the rest of your life, unless you pull the ripcord and stop.

I'm not talking about the useful conversations between friends who are trying to figure out what a problem is and then working to solve it. Commiserating is very different: it's talking about your problems, making excuses for why you can't solve them, then having your girlfriend validate your lack of action.

Sitting around with your friends and talking about how hard everything is, or how you deserve to engage in self-destructive behaviors because you've earned it, or putting yourself down to make everyone else feel more comfortable — aka, commiserating — has got to stop.

Commiserating wrecks your confidence and keeps you stuck in mediocrity. But we fall prey to it because it feels easier to make excuses instead of taking responsibility, and our friends validate us because they haven't achieved the results they want either.

I'm not trying to sound harsh — I've done it, too. So have all of us. But I know you want results and a different way of life that comes with those results. And you deserve that life. You're a lot stronger than you think, and you're more capable than you give yourself credit for. But commiserating with other people about your problems instead of getting busy solving them will keep you stuck.

162

You deserve a lot better, and a huge step in the right direction is to quit having these useless, negative, success-destroying conversations. Also, the more you repeat false truths, the more your brain will look for ways for you to back them up — which equals frequent binges, half-assed workouts, and more excuses. And don't forget that whatever words you speak aloud have a lot more power than those that exist only in your mind.

Justifying your lack of progress in any area means that you will continue never making progress. And making excuses prevents you from taking responsibility for your life. If you keep doing this, you will keep making yourself powerless — when you are anything but.

Strategies

Say no. It's very simple. Stop spending time with people who want to commiserate. It feels hard to say no, because women are conditioned to not be "rude" and to make everyone feel good. (Everyone but ourselves, that is.)

You don't have to cut people off or insult them, but you can say in the nicest way possible that you have other plans. And you don't have to say what those other plans are. You don't have to make up stories or explain why you can't join them. A simple "No thanks, I can't" is enough. Refuse to participate in these kinds of conversations.

Just saying no without explaining yourself is liberating and builds your confidence in an amazing way — and you can use all that confidence to go achieve your goals instead of sitting around talking about how impossible they are to achieve.

Find a new friend. You have at least one success-minded friend. Call that person today and make a plan to get together and strategize how you're going to achieve your weight-loss goal. Enlist her to keep you accountable and help you work toward its achievement. Go walking together, go eat a healthy dinner with her, go get a green juice instead of a glass of wine.

People who are positive and uplifting are exactly who you need to spend time with if you're determined to achieve any kind of goal. You want to hear as much encouragement and have as many motivating conversations as possible. And if you feel uncomfortable calling someone and talking about your goals with that person, remember that growth-minded people don't make excuses, never laugh at other people's goals, and certainly don't convince them to not try.

Recommit to your goals. If you don't keep your goals in the forefront of your mind, they'll vanish into thin air. And don't forget that you need to write them down — daily.

The fastest way to make sure your dreams die is to talk yourself out of achieving them by commiserating about how hard they are to achieve with people who have no goals of their own.

But it's not enough to only not engage in these kinds of conversations — you have to actively recommit to your goals. Committing to them over and over again reinforces your motivation to continue taking actions toward their achievement. And it also makes the commiserating conversations highly unappealing and therefore less likely to occur.

Believing in the Magic Pill

The Magic Pill doesn't exist. And as long as you keep trying to find it, you'll stay stuck.

You keep looking for it because you feel desperate. But the reason you feel desperate is because you've been trying diet after diet, which all are some form of the Magic Pill — none of them ever deliver what they promise, and they all result in failure.

Ironically, your faith in a diet and its promise of magical map that you can follow to the perfect life is what keeps you from succeeding on it. That's because by being fully swept up in this fantasy and believing in it so wholeheartedly, you make yourself helpless. That means you never access your inner power to make your own changes.

But if you reject this fantasy and start making slow, steady changes, your confidence will grow, and with it your power. Then your desperation will evaporate. The more action you take, the less desperate you become, and pretty soon there's no need for the Magic Pill.

Once you put all that misplaced faith in yourself, you'll start succeeding . . . and also realize that there's no such thing as failure. The true magic is you deciding you're going to take control and start making changes — and the power you feel from that is what makes it all happen.

Strategies

Refuse to be sucked in. Anytime you hear about a new diet, block it out. See it for what it is. No matter how different it looks on the surface, remember that at their core, diets are all the same. And that's why none of them work.

Change the channel, close the browser, use whatever mantra you have to block it out! It's messier and way more scary to go it alone, but remember that's what builds confidence and power, which is how you get real results. You know the truth, and you're not going to fall for that anymore.

Don't commiserate. Refer to the previous section. Commiserating with people, putting yourself down, talking about how fat you are and how awful you look, sharing sarcastic memes about your wine baby — don't do it. It seems harmless, but all of it adds up to a collective lack of confidence — which makes you more susceptible to the next diet.

Listen to the talk, but don't absorb it. You don't have to be rude, but don't buy in. There's no magic pill,

Take massive action. Massive action transforms you into a completely different human being and obliterates all obstacles in your path. It makes you feel decisive, in control, and capable — and therefore less likely to feel desperate for a magic pill.

This doesn't just apply to weight loss. Take massive action in every area of your life, because it spills over — and it becomes a habit to take control, get busy, and do something. You'll start feeling less like a helpless victim and more like a strong confident woman who's capable of not just losing weight but of creating the life she deserves to live.

Upgrade Your Environment

Environment is the invisible hand
that shapes human behavior.

— *James Clear*

Your environment is absolutely critical to your success at losing weight — or to the achievement of any goal.

To put it more accurately, taking control of your environment is what's critical to your success. Unfortunately, not only do most people not take control of their environments, they don't even notice them.

If you don't actively take control of your environment, it will silently prevent you from achieving your goals. Let that sink in for a minute. If you don't make a concerted effort to construct an environment that is set up for your success, you're going to fail.

The worst part about this is that women tend to blame themselves for not having enough willpower, not being dedicated enough, or lacking the motivation to achieve their weight-loss goal. When in fact, a huge part of their failure is that their environment is working against them. It's like trying to climb Mt. Everest with a sack of cement on your back.

But that's only half of the analogy. Having someone take the weight off your back, although extremely helpful, is not all there is. What if someone also gave you a pair of brand new running shoes and guided you to the summit?

That's what proactively setting your environment up will do for you. Not only will you remove all the obstacles from your path, you will construct it so that your success is inevitable and far easier to achieve.

So why do so many people leave out this part of the process? Well, first of all, they're not aware of how strongly linked environment is to results. But the main reason people neglect to set their environments up for success is that they no longer even see what's around them.

You're so used to looking at your current surroundings that it's become like white noise. You can't see it. But sadly it's almost certain that your environment contains all kinds of barriers to your success — and even worse, it actually pushes you to fail.

I'd be willing to bet that if I came to your house and looked around, I would be able to find at least ten huge barriers that are keeping you from losing weight — and I'd be able to give you a hundred small modifications you could make to eliminate them.

Even if you're a type A, clutter-hating neat freak, I could find things that are getting in the way of your success. And without a doubt I could give you even more changes you could make to make your goal easier to achieve.

I like to call your environment your secret weight-loss weapon. And the best part is that you already have the weapon — you're just not using it to your advantage. But if you don't proactively use it, it will passively sabotage you.

So it's tempting to think, "Oh that's a really cool concept. I'll get around to fixing my environment at some point." But remember, it's already working — whether you notice it or not. And if the results you're currently getting aren't the results you want, it's almost certain your environment isn't set up properly.

The good news is that it's super easy to change your environment, because there are infinite ways to change it. And the really good news is that one small change has the potential to add up to massive results, because each change you make sets off a chain reaction to other positive changes. And just like with your habits, you start to get exponential results.

How it works

Your environment has a powerful influence on what you think, how you feel, and what you do. And when it comes to your eating habits, your environment may be pushing you to say "who cares" and eat whatever's in front of you.

What you look at shapes your thoughts, and your thoughts dictate what you do. So if you're looking at a cluttered kitchen that has a fridge full of expired foods, you're probably not going to be motivated to cook a healthy meal — or anything, for that matter. If your kitchen is constantly a mess, you're probably going to feel exhausted or frustrated, which means you're more likely to binge on something.

Also, if your environment is working against you, you'll waste a lot of energy trying to overcome it — energy you would rather use to keep yourself on track with your habit-changing efforts. Taking control of your environment can help you more than all your other healthy behaviors combined because it affects every single one of them.

According to success author James Clear, "Environment is the invisible hand that shapes human behavior." This quote nicely sums up two critical points: 1) Your environment powerfully affects your actions, and 2) you don't realize it's happening. Because you're so used to seeing what's around you, you can't see how your environment is sabotaging you.

So let's see exactly how this works. Habits are nothing more than your brain's way of simplifying movements so that it can use its energy for more complicated tasks or to problem-solve.

For example, you no longer have to think about all the left and right turns you need to take on your way home from dropping your kids off at school. You've done this so many times that your brain has you on autopilot. But there was a point in time that you did need directions. However, after driving the route over and over again, your brain memorized the way to go, and now you get there automatically. It's habitual.

Any habit you've developed is because you've done it so many times that it's become ingrained in your neural network. Actually, that's exactly how habits become habits: new neural pathways become established so that your neurons fire more easily down those paths.

If you've conditioned yourself to have certain thoughts over and over again — like "This always happens to me" or "Look at the bright side" (way better!) — you'll keep strengthening the tendency to think those thoughts, because of your brain's ability to adapt itself to make them automatic. And then it can help you more effectively when you're figuring out how to do something more difficult, like learn to speak a foreign language.

Your environment pushes you to engage in behaviors repeatedly, and eventually your brain makes them habits. It's estimated that your habits are responsible for 40% of the actions you take daily,[2] so if your environment is shaping your habits and your habits cause you to

---

[2] Science Daily. How we form habits, change existing ones. August 8, 2014. https://www.sciencedaily.com/releases/2014/08/140808111931.htm. Accessed May 14, 2020.

take nearly half of the actions you take on a daily basis, you can get the idea of how critical it is to take control of it.

Your environment makes you feel a certain way, these feelings create thoughts, those thoughts create actions, and those actions create habits. And your habits create results.

Let's look at two examples. Let's say you are a smoker and you want to quit. You decide that Monday is the day, and you're totally committed and motivated. You're ready to finally get rid of this destructive habit, and you decide that nothing is going to stop you.

You wake up on Monday, and while you're in your living room having coffee, you notice the dirty ash tray on your coffee table. Then you look for your car keys and stumble on a pack of cigarettes you forgot to throw out. You go to work and take your usual coffee break with your coworkers, and they all smoke a cigarette while you chat. You go home after work, and when you walk in, the smell of smoke is overpowering. Your furniture smells like smoke, your clothes smell like smoke, your bed smells like smoke. The evidence of your smoking habit is everywhere — stray packs of cigarettes, ash trays you forgot to get rid of, and the smell of smoke permeating your home. How successful do you think you'll be to quit smoking with all of these environmental factors in place? Not very.

Or let's use an example of the kind all-or-nothing health overall that's familiar to anyone who's been on a diet. Let's say you're going to eliminate sugar and alcohol for an entire week, and you're going to work out every single day.

On day one, your alarm doesn't go off, and you accidentally oversleep. The first thing you see when you jump out of bed is the two loads of laundry you didn't get done over the weekend. Then you head to your kitchen, and it looks like a bomb went off.

Now you're running late, you're totally stressed out, and your kids are behind schedule. You hurriedly pack their lunches and scarf down a few Oreos while you're doing it. You're already late, so you don't have time to work out. You promise yourself you'll get back on track tomorrow.

While you're cleaning up your kitchen later, you stumble across some candy and grab a few pieces. You've already missed your workout and had some cookies, so what difference does it make? You were going to clean your house while the kids were at school, but now you're in a sugar crash so you collapse onto the couch and watch television.

By the time your kids get home, you're completely demoralized from your failures, and now you're irritated, too. They make even more of a mess, you lose your patience and yell at them — and now you're not only going to have that glass of wine but you feel like drinking the whole bottle.

Both of these scenarios could have been prevented entirely by a few strategic environmental changes. Notice that the individual stumbling blocks aren't necessarily deal-breakers on their own. But when added together, they create destruction.

So even if you commit to doing everything right, with the wrong environment you will fail. No amount of motivation or willpower in the world is enough to overcome your environment.

The research

Research backs up how influential your environment is on your actions and habits. Let's look specifically at the research involving the relationship between the environment and your health behaviors.

It's well-known in the marketing industry how product placement affects the buying habits of consumers. Incredible sums of money are spent on figuring out exactly how companies should place their products in order to get people to buy them.

For example, grocery stores place items they want you to buy in the middle of the store and at eye level. They know which items you frequently purchase or need most often, so those are placed in the back of the store or on lower shelves. If they know you're going to buy it or need it regularly, they know you'll actively go looking for it.

For example, they put the milk and eggs all the way in the back of the store, because they know you came there specifically to get those things. The more expensive or not-necessary items — like high-end olive oil or fancy organic potato chips — are placed in the middle of the store at eye level, where you're more likely to see them as you walk past them on the way to get your milk. That way, you're more likely to buy them. And marketing research shows that you do.

In one study of the marketing practices of grocery stores, research showed that when stores doubled the size of their carts, shoppers bought on average 40% more products. Also, grocery stores are designed to get you to travel down each aisle. They know that if they strategically place displays at the beginning of an aisle you're more likely to go down that aisle — but they also break up longer aisles so that you don't avoid them for fear of being "trapped."[3]

I'm sure you never think about any of this as you make your run to the store every week, but you're being environmentally influenced to buy as much as your grocery store can possibly sell you.

Academic research focused on eating behaviors also shows how environmental factors heavily influence what you choose to eat and how much of it you do. In one laboratory study of portion sizes, participants were offered three different serving sizes of mac and cheese, and researchers calculated the amount of food consumed. The people who chose the largest portion size ate 30% more food than the ones who chose the smallest portion.[4]

---

[3] Today. Supermarkets wage war for your dollars. January 27, 2001. https://www.today.com/news/supermarkets-wage-war-your-dollars-wbna41259243. Accessed May 14, 2020.

[4] Rolls BJ. The Supersizing of America. Nutr Today 2003 Mar-Apr;38(2):42-53.

In another study that looked at the relationship between utensil size and amount of food consumed, participants who used smaller forks were more likely to eat less than those who used a larger fork. But, interestingly, this only held true for the participants who ate in a home environment as opposed to those who ate in a restaurant environment.

Participants who ate in a restaurant ate more food when using a smaller rather than a larger fork. Researchers hypothesized that this was a result of perceived value — people wanted to get the value they felt they deserved in exchange for paying for the food.[5] This difference highlights how different environmental factors influence people in different and sometimes divergent ways.

In another study, researchers who wanted to improve the food and beverage choices of hospital staff and patrons placed bottled water in baskets at the checkout counter of the cafeteria. When they did this, bottled water consumption increased by 25%.[6]

In another study of the influence of environment on women's health behaviors, researchers studied the kitchens of 500 women. They asked all women to describe what was on their kitchen counters, and they visited the actual kitchens of 200 of these women and took photographs. They also assessed the BMI — or body mass index, a measure of obesity based on height and weight — of all the women.[7]

What they found was fascinating. Women who were in the normal BMI range were more likely than women who were classified as

[5] Mishra A, Mishra H, Masters TM. The influence of bite size on quantity of food consumed: a field study. J Consumer Res 2012;38(5):791-5.

[6] Thorndike AN, Sonnenberg L, Riis J, Barraclough S, Levy DE. A 2-Phase labeling and choice architecture Intervention to improve healthy food and beverage choices. Am J Public Health 2012;102(3):527-33.

[7] Wansink B, et al. Slim by design: kitchen counter correlates of obesity. Health Educ Behav 2016;43(5):552-8.

overweight to have a bowl of fruit on their counters and to not have chips or crackers on the counter or anywhere in sight. Not only that, women whose *only* countertop item was a bowl of fruit had a lower BMI than all the other participants.

In addition, women who kept cereal on the counter weighed an average of 21 pounds more than those who kept their cereal in the pantry, and women who kept soda in visible locations in their kitchens — whether it was regular soda or diet soda — weighed an average of 26 more pounds than those who kept it out of sight.

It's important to note than none of these studies were the "gold standard" of research — randomized, double-blind, or placebo-controlled, meaning that participants are randomly assigned to one of two groups, neither the researchers nor the participants knows which ones they were assigned to, and there is a neutral variable that is used for comparison to the variable being studied. All of which means that the results of these kinds of studies are more likely to be accurate.

However, the anecdotal evidence is convincing enough for me to confidently conclude that environment has a definite effect on your behavior — and that if you modify it in your favor, it can help you instead of sabotage you.

What it looks like in action

So what does all this research look like in action? The clearest takeaway is that certain environmental changes can have a dramatic effect on your eating habits and, subsequently, your weight.

If you wanted to get specific, eating with a smaller fork, putting cereal or crackers or soda out of sight and off your countertop, and placing healthier items like fruit or water on your countertop would be the obvious changes to make.

But think about why that is. The common denominator in all these changes is the use of barriers. You're putting barriers in place to prevent you from engaging in bad habits, and you're removing the barriers that keep you from engaging in good habits.

In the kitchen counter study, the women who put their cereal and soda on their counters weighed more — significantly more — than the women who couldn't see all of those things on a daily basis. Because they could see those items, they (presumably) were more likely to eat those items. There wasn't a barrier that kept them from snacking on chips when they were hungry or grabbing a Coke when they were thirsty. They had no barriers between them and these bad habits.

But the women who had to open a cabinet or walk into their pantry to get these things were (again, presumably) less likely to mindlessly eat or drink them. (I have to say "presumably" since you can't prove any of this. I guess it's possible that the reason all the women who kept their soda in the pantry weighed less was because they were all marathon runners, but I doubt it.)

The women who weighed the least not only didn't have the unhealthy items constantly in their faces, but they also had healthy items where they could consistently see them. In other words, having the fruit on the counter made it easier to eat that fruit. Maybe this is why they weighed so much less than the other women — because they had a barrier to the bad behavior in place and they also had no barrier to the good behavior. No chips on the counter makes it harder to snack on them, and having fruit on the counter makes it easier to eat. Those two in combination added up to weighing less — a lot less.

In this scenario, the barrier to the bad behaviors of snacking on chips and drinking soda was nothing more than having to open up a cabinet or taking a few steps toward the pantry. And the barrier to eating fruit that was removed was not having to take the additional step of opening up the refrigerator to take it out. All it took was a few additional seconds or expending a small amount of energy to keep the women from acting on an impulse. And by not having to spend time overthinking whether they should have an apple or something less healthy, they chose the apple instead.

In the other studies, putting bottled water at the checkout where customers could see it made them more likely to buy it. And using a smaller fork and making a smaller serving made it less likely for participants to overeat.

But let's go one layer deeper and look at what's really going on. If you use barriers this way what happens is that these small decisions are being made for you — you don't have to think about what to do. Therefore, you don't have to use willpower to not make the wrong decisions, and you don't have to motivate yourself to actively make the right ones.

These tiny decisions that you make all day, every day, add up to massive results. Think about that: the women who kept chips and soda where they could see it weighed roughly 20 pounds more than the women who didn't. You can't prove that they weighed more because of this, but I'm pretty sure that out of 500 women this may have had something to do with it. If all you have to do is make the investment of putting away the chips and leaving some fruit on the counter to get this kind of a return, I think it's worth it, don't you?

Imagine if you put all of these environmental changes in place. If you started eating with a smaller fork and putting your food on a smaller plate, you kept all of the chips, crackers, soda, and sweets out of sight, and you kept your countertop empty save for a bowl of fruit and some bottled water — you could instantly and dramatically increase your odds of losing weight. You wouldn't have to throw everything out and buy all new food, you wouldn't have to gear yourself up for a week of using willpower to try "not to," and you wouldn't have to force yourself to eat healthy.

What a massive relief. And with the elimination of all that negative energy, you'd have creative energy to effortlessly do something inspiring or fun that makes you feel good — instead of feeling defeated and like the only thing that would make you feel better is to eat something. Not only that, having your environment help you make the right choices consistently means that over time you effortlessly form new habits.

What you want to do is eliminate the need to think — you want to "de-think" your environment. You want to insert barriers to bad behaviors and remove the barriers to good behaviors. You want to eliminate the need for willpower and motivation. You want to set your environment up so that it makes decisions for you.

Ideally you should do this for every environment you are in on a regular basis, but there's no environment more important to your success at losing weight than your kitchen. The next how-to steps can be applied to your closet, your bedroom, your office, even your car. But I'm going to focus in particular on your kitchen — since that's where all the food is!

How to do it

1. Purge it. Clutter creates overwhelm, and feeling overwhelmed leads to making bad decisions. If you eliminate the clutter from your kitchen, you're going to feel lighter and less stressed, so you'll be less likely to binge eat.

Take everything out of your cabinets, drawers, and pantry. Organize it into 1) I use it all the time, 2) I use it some of the time, and 3) I hardly ever use it. Start with the things you hardly ever use. Unless it's a family heirloom or something of significant emotional value, get rid of it! Even if it's serving platters or fancy salt and pepper shakers you got for your wedding, please do yourself a favor and give it away.

For the things you use only some of the time, your goal is to get rid of half of it. Many of the items in this pile probably fall into the "one day" category. Maybe one day you'll use that margarita pitcher you bought when you were in college or that jar of peach marmalade you got for Christmas five years ago. Probably not. If it's something you really love that will inspire you to do something fun or try a new dish, keep it. But you know which items are just taking up space and need to go. You're not allowed to feel guilty or wasteful. Be ruthless!

For the perishable items, throw out anything expired, about to expire, that has been open for a month or more (sugar, flour), or that you know you'll never use (hot sauce, jelly). Things you use all the time you will obviously keep.

Don't try to do this all in one day. Take it one cabinet, drawer, or area at a time. Make it fun, and enjoy the feeling of making your life a whole lot lighter. A good tip for this phase is to set a timer, so you don't overthink it.

2. Clean it out. After you purge each area, wipe it down with vinegar and hot water. I don't like using chemical sprays like 409 because I don't like anything scented, but if that doesn't bother you, go right ahead. I also like to get a dustbuster and vacuum it out first — I even do that in my fridge and freezer because I'm psycho like that. Clean and sanitize everything.

3. Get organized. Your goal is for everything to have a home and for you to be able to see most of everything. You don't want stuff hiding behind other items, because if you can't see it, you won't use it. (If you can't make this happen, you probably didn't purge enough.) Group similar items together and nest items if possible (bowls, Tupperware).

Buy containers and to make it easier to separate, store, and access everything. Buy some bamboo drawer dividers for your silverware, vacuum-sealed containers for items like flour and sugar that are messy after opening, and stackable drawers for things like sponges and drain stoppers under your sink. Buy all new Tupperware, and get rid of all that mismatched crap.

You don't have to spend a ton of money, unless you want to — you can go all the way from Target to Williams Sonoma, depending on how much you want to invest.

4. Set it up. Here's where your kitchen starts making decisions for you. Set your kitchen up so that the foods you want to eat are at eye level or out where you can see them. Put olive oil on the counter so you're inspired to cook, and of course put a bowl of fruit on the counter! Put items that you don't want to eat or that you want to eat less out of sight, put them in harder-to-reach areas, and group them together, if possible. Put the chocolate on a higher shelf, put your kids' snacks all on one shelf or in a big snack drawer.

Get a system going in your refrigerator. Group all similar items together, which you probably already do, but also make them flow in and out easily. Adhere to the first-in, first-out procedure — if you buy a carton of milk because you're about to run out, put the new one behind the one that's about to be done. Arrange fruits and vegetables so that the ones that are about to expire are in front, ready to use. Eliminate the need to rummage through a bunch of stuff to find what you're looking for.

Put the healthier items you want to eat right in the middle of the fridge where those are the first things you see. Even if you're just getting something for your kids, it's a reminder of your commitment to eat healthy just to see all the fruits and vegetables you just bought, staring you in the face every time you open the doors. I like to put the foods I'm planning on eating that day all on one shelf — and when I've eaten everything on that shelf, I'm done for the day. Line up bottles of water on one shelf. And, again, I know I'm a freak, but I swear if you turn all the labels the same way, it makes you feel even more organized and in control!

180

Get a meal magnet for your refrigerator, and plan out two or three days of meals. Have a dedicated sticky note pad where you keep a running grocery list. It sounds basic, and it is, but just having a spot to jot down what you need as soon as you think of it is one more thing you took off your mental plate. It gets out of control fast when you don't pay attention to these kinds of details. Trying to remember everything because you don't have somewhere to write it all down means you forget things, you feel stressed out at the store and buy a bunch stuff you don't need, you don't have what you need to cook that meal you planned on, and you say screw it and binge on whatever's randomly lying around — probably something unhealthy you had in plain sight out on your countertop.

Every time you take the trash out, weed stuff out of your fridge. This keeps you on top of things and prevents your kitchen from getting out of flow. If you know no one's going to eat that leftover pizza, take it out with the trash — even if it's still good! Don't keep things that you know won't get eaten. If you're just waiting until it goes bad until you throw it out, it's taking up space in your fridge and creating more mental weight for you to deal with.

5. Make it pretty! You want to feel good in your kitchen. Making your kitchen a space you want to be in is so important if you want to have a healthy relationship with food. Remember, if you want to have healthy eating habits, you absolutely must cook, at least some of the time. And if being in your kitchen makes you feel burdened or stressed out, you will never cook.

After you get everything cleaned out and organized, take some time to make your kitchen beautiful. It doesn't take much: buy some fresh flowers or an herb plant, light a candle, get an Alexa and play classical music. Take a few pieces of the china and crystal you hardly ever use — and use it! Hang some of your kids' artwork, put an attractive cookbook on the counter, get a colorful glass bowl to put your fruit in. Whatever makes you feel peaceful, creative, or joyful, do it.

Take absolute control in every area of your kitchen, make healthy foods flow easily in and out, and make your kitchen a place you want to spend time in — not somewhere that makes you feel like cooking is a chore or where you have to summon all kinds of willpower not to eat.

If you want a more detailed guide to set your kitchen up properly, I've created Your Ultimate Weight-Loss Kitchen, which will show you step by step how to do it. You can get it at camillemartinrd.com/shop.

It's not just your house

Remember that your environment isn't just limited to your physical surroundings — it includes your mental, emotional, and social environments, too.

Be careful what you read when you're surfing the web. Pay close attention to what you watch on television. I know by saying this I may make myself sound completely ignorant, but I never, ever watch the news. I don't watch it, and I don't read about it. It's mostly negative, doomsday stuff, and I want every piece of information that filters through my brain to lift me up and make me feel good — not like the world is coming to an end an there's no hope for humanity.

I'm confident that if there's something I need to know about, it will appear as one of the banner headlines, and seeing that will keep me more than informed. Inundating yourself with horrible and upsetting stories about child abductions, animal abuse, and political rants and tirades infiltrates your brain and dramatically affects your mood — even if you think it doesn't. And your mood and how you feel dictates what you do.

Read an inspiring book that helps you develop a new skill or motivates you to create something. Take a walk. Call a friend. Keep your mindset free from negativity and make yourself feel as much joy as you possibly can.

Speaking of calling a friend, make sure it's a positive friend. Your social environment is everything if you want to achieve a goal or grow in any way as a human being. Remember not to commiserate with people about how hard it is to lose weight or how horrible life is. Absolutely refuse to engage in political discussions — in my experience, these go absolutely nowhere and do nothing but wind everyone up for no reason. It's my experience that nobody wins a cocktail party political debate.

Cultivate friendships with people who are interested in life and in creating something or lifting people up. This isn't Pollyanna stuff — it's critical to your happiness not to spend time with toxic people. There's a popular saying that you become the average of the five people you hang out with the most. Whether that's true or not, and I think it is, it's a terrifying possibility if you spend a large part of your time with negative people.

You don't have to cut people out of your life, but say no as often as you can and as nicely as you can. And you'll be amazed at how these people will start eliminating themselves once you commit to becoming the best version of yourself. Negative people don't like being around people who won't join in with them or who have goals, so they'll automatically go looking for someone else to drag down.

––––––

You want to set up your eating environment to make engaging in healthy habits practically automatic. You don't have to keep using willpower to make changes or endure the incessant inner debate of should I or shouldn't I. You can make it a whole lot easier to make progress and also create lots of positive energy that can be used more productively.

There are hundreds of small ways to modify your environment, and every time you make a small change, that small win spills over to other areas. And any one of these tiny changes has the potential to set off a cascade of other changes, leading to massive results.

Just the act of making these kinds of environmental improvements makes you feel confident and in control, which is one of the reasons this tactic is so powerful. You need to feel confident and in control if you want to make changes that stick and ultimately transform your life.

But most important, remember that your environment powerfully affects you and everything you do, whether you realize it or not. It can be an invisible supporter or a silent destroyer — it's up to you. Take charge of it, and use it to your advantage.

A Larger Goal

You are never too old to set another goal

or to dream a new dream.

— C. S. Lewis

Do you wake up every morning, consumed with a cherished dream you have for yourself, thinking of the steps you'll take that day in order to make it a reality? My guess is the answer would be a resounding no. My guess is that you don't even allow yourself to have a dream, much less have it converted into a goal you're actively working toward. And if you bought this book, my guess is that the only goal you've truly had for a very long time is to lose weight.

When was the last time you allowed yourself to even have a dream? The kind of dream I'm talking about is the one that flashes across your mind while you're in a quiet moment walking on the beach, and for a split second you allow yourself to go there. The kind of dream when you think to yourself, "Wouldn't it be amazing if . . .?"

Sadly, these dreams only last for a fleeting, enthralling second — until you snap yourself back to reality and kill it before it can even take a shallow breath.

Why do we do this? Why do we not even allow ourselves to contemplate something amazing for our lives? Why are we so quick to believe that these dreams aren't possible or that we're even worthy of having them?

Part of the reason is that we've dumbed ourselves down for so long, wasting years of our lives trying to lose weight, that we've lost sight of who we are and who we're capable of becoming. That plus also spending years of our lives doing everything for other people and doing very little for ourselves. We've gotten so far away from the dreamers we used to be that we've forgotten we had dreams at all.

But having a dream for your life isn't just for super-accomplished people. It's not just for the Bill Gateses and the Madonnas of the world . . . it's for you, too. And it's not just something indulgent that you do while jogging on the beach — it's something you should actively do on a daily basis.

Having a larger goal is essential for a fulfilling existence on this earth. And if you're not entirely convinced that a big goal is for you, at least consider this: having a really big goal can help you lose weight.

Why you need a larger goal

According to psychologist Abraham Maslow, human beings have needs that must be met in order to thrive. He developed a well-known hierarchy to describe these needs, which start with the most fundamental physiological needs, like food, water, and shelter. He hypothesized that once these basic needs are met, people travel up the hierarchy through emotional and self-esteem–related needs until they reach the top, where you find the ultimate human need: self-actualization. In other words, the need to reach one's fullest potential.

186

I'm assuming that you have a home to live in, emotional connections with other people, and a certain amount of self-esteem. So if it feels like something is missing, it's highly likely that you're not attempting to live to your fullest potential.

It's challenging to identify this. You would probably argue with me that anything is missing from your life. But if you have that nagging feeling that your life was supposed to be more exciting than this, then what you need is a goal to work toward. You need to re-engage with life and remind yourself what you're capable of.

To clarify, I'm not saying that close, connected relationships with your husband and children and making sacrifices for them isn't both necessary and beautiful, because it is. But you also need to live a fulfilled life on your own. And here's the important point: these two things don't have to be mutually exclusive. The need for self-actualization is a basic human need. It's not selfish.

In fact, having a purpose for your life that has nothing to do with those around you makes you better able to support them. You become a better partner, mother, employee, and friend the more you're working toward your fullest potential. The excitement and enthusiasm that come with having a big dream and working toward it spill over to all your relationships and infuse them with that positive energy, making them stronger and better.

If this is still hard to wholeheartedly accept, think of it this way: if all you do all day is think about losing weight and you spend a significant amount of time constantly dieting and failing, over and over again, this negative energy also spills over into those relationships — in the form of frustration, impatience, resentment, and disconnection.

So I strongly believe that having a dream and a goal for your life is necessary not only for you, but also for everyone you have a relationship with.

Having a larger goal makes you feel enthusiastic and excited about your life. It gives you something to look forward to every day. It gives your life purpose and meaning and makes you feel hopeful about the future. It gives you a sense of what's possible for your life.

And when you set a big goal and start working to achieve it, you build confidence. You start to see what you're capable of — and realize it's a whole lot more than you've been giving yourself credit for.

You'll probably easily achieve your first big goal and clearly see that you should have set a bigger one. Then you'll keep right on going. The best part is that there's no failure, because the only real failure is not trying at all.

How it will help you lose weight

Trying to lose weight is a negative-focused goal. You're focused on trying to get rid of something, which puts you in a resistant frame of mind. And, as I already discussed, wanting to lose weight focuses you directly on something you hate, which defeats you from the outset.

Again, having a larger, more exciting goal puts you in a creative state that makes taking action automatic and fun, as opposed to something you're forcing yourself to do. It makes you proactive instead of reactive — it takes you from trying "not to" to actively taking steps, gaining momentum, and consistently moving forward.

When your only goal is to lose weight, your life starts to close in on itself. If you keep feeling like a failure over and over again, your whole life becomes a chore. If you feel like a failure, it's an effort to do even the most basic daily tasks. You feel stuck and stagnant in your life, which makes you feel like "Is this all there is?"

But when you have something to get up every day to work toward, something that excites you, everything else becomes effortless. You have more energy, so cooking, cleaning, car-pooling, errand-running, and working are easier. When these things become easier and you get them done faster and more efficiently, you feel super successful instead of lethargic and unmotivated.

This feeling of accomplishment makes you take better care of yourself automatically. And working out and eating healthy will become enjoyable instead of something you "have" to do.

Your newfound creative energy will make you want to take a long walk with your dog instead of forcing yourself to the gym. Instead of willing yourself not to binge eat your frozen meal, you'll be in your kitchen, planning the healthy dinner you're going to cook. And you'll start doing more self-care activities, like meditating, reading, journaling, and hydrating — because you'll value yourself and your health instead of hating your body and trying to fix yourself from the outside in.

You won't have to use willpower to stop yourself from eating, because you won't be thinking about eating at all. You'll be so busy working toward your big goal that losing weight isn't even on your radar anymore.

Bigger is better

So now that you are convinced (I hope) of the necessity of having a bigger goal, let's talk about how to set one. More specifically, let's talk about how not to set one.

One of the biggest problems with setting a big goal is that most people don't go big enough. This is especially true if you've spent years of your life feeling like a failure from never having lost weight. You feel like "How am I going to do that if I can't even lose ten pounds?"

But it's critically important to push through that feeling and go ahead and set the big goal anyway. Forget about whether you think you can actually achieve it. The truth is that you should set a goal that seems just out of reach, and here's why.

A goal that isn't awe-inspiring and that doesn't feel a little scary doesn't generate the motivation required to see it through. If you set a too-small goal, you don't get the feeling of excitement that pushes you to go after it. The butterflies-in-your-stomach feeling is exactly what you want.

The energy you generate by setting a huge goal is what will make you bound out of bed in the morning and take action. The anticipation and enthusiasm you feel from having the goal are what push you to take the steps necessary for its achievement. A goal that doesn't truly excite you doesn't create enough energy to make you feel like doing much of anything.

The reason people don't set big goals is because they're afraid they don't have what it takes to achieve them. But it's in the pursuit of a big goal that you become the kind of person that *can* achieve it. And that's the whole point! It's about living to your fullest potential, and if you have nothing to work toward, you'll never see what that potential is.

Don't be afraid to set a really big goal. Even if you don't get all the way across the finish line, there is no failure. The only failure is not trying at all.

You don't have to tell anyone about your goal. In fact, I would keep it to yourself at the outset. It's too easy for people to crush it before it gets a chance to come to life. I've found that people don't discourage you from going after a goal or a dream to be unkind or unsupportive. They want to protect you from being disappointed. And it's also possible that they gave up on their dreams a long time ago, so it's easier for them to discourage you than to watch you go for it and make it real.

And if the people close to you are afraid this new big goal is going to take you away from them and all the other responsibilities you have, remind them that becoming more of who you really are only makes you better equipped to take care of everyone else.

Keep in mind that what seems like a huge goal for you might look super easy for someone else. It's a certainty that it will. But remember that something that's effortless for you looks unachievable for someone else.

Only you know which is which. If running a 5K seems completely out of reach, then make that your big goal. And if it's a marathon, let that be it.

Also, choose a goal that's yours. Don't set a goal because you think it's what someone else would pick or that would impress the people around you. And especially don't pick a goal based on whether it would threaten them or take you away from them.

If you want to go back to school and get a nursing degree, make that your goal. If you want to go on an archeological dig, set the goal. If your dream is to start an online business selling jewelry, set the goal! Remember, it doesn't matter if you think you can actually achieve it.

You want to set a goal that seems just out of reach. If it doesn't give you that internal spark, go back to the drawing board, because it's not big enough!

Fundamentals of setting a big goal

The first thing you may be wondering is what kind of goal you should set. Again, the two most important requirements of your big goal are 1) it generates tremendous excitement and 2) you're setting it for you, not based on what anyone else thinks or how it will affect them. Remember: this is all about you.

The next section is about the nuts-and-bolts process to set your goal, but there are some other fundamental things to keep in mind when setting your goal.

As I just said, the biggest deterrent to setting a big goal is your belief that you won't be able to achieve it. This belief may stem from feeling that you're actually incapable of doing it (running a

191

marathon, starring in a movie, being a motivational speaker) or that it's logistically unrealistic to do (taking time away from your family to get a second degree or devoting resources to starting a business). It can feel almost impossible to even decide on something because your "reality" stops you before you even get started.

The way to overcome this is to use visualization. Whatever goal you choose, you want to spend every stray moment of your days picturing yourself with the dream already achieved. There is evidence that doing this makes you more likely to achieve the goal and for it to happen faster.

For example, professional athletes use this technique to enhance their performance, have an edge over their competitors, and increase their chances of winning a game or a gold medal. They envision the event down to the last detail — even imagining the roar of the crowd or the interview they will give after winning. Olympic athletes tell stories of seeing their opponents at the starting line with their eyes closed, performing the actions they'll take while competing. And they spend a significant amount of money on sports psychologists, who assist the athletes with these kinds of techniques.[8]

Envision yourself taking the steps necessary to achieve the goal, and especially imagine yourself once the goal is achieved. See yourself succeeding in a big way. Picture yourself standing at the podium giving your speech, on stage receiving your diploma, in the foreign country speaking the language. Imagine what you're wearing, what you're saying, what's around you — down to the smallest detail.

Intense visualization builds tremendous momentum that you'll then act on, making your goal begin to come to life and the chances

---

[8] Clarey C. Olympians use imagery as mental training. New York Times. February 22, 2014. https://www.nytimes.com/2014/02/23/sports/olympics/olympians-use-imagery-as-mental-training.html. Accessed May 14, 2020.

of you achieving it exponentially higher. It also gives you a rush of excitement to see yourself living your dream, and this excitement will color everything else you do for the rest of the day.

I already mentioned the importance of writing your dream down, so I won't repeat all of it here. But once you visualize yourself achieving your goal, you must write it down at least once every day to keep it at the forefront of your mind. Also, don't forget to write it in the present tense: "I am a New York Times #1 bestselling author," "I am fluent in Italian," "I am a triathlete."

The final element of setting a big goal is to back it up with a larger purpose. Having a really good "why" gives you even more motivation to stick with it and consistently work toward its achievement.

If you want to become a bestselling author, maybe it's because you want to help people in some way. Even if you want to write fiction, your "why" is to entertain people and bring them joy. If you want to speak a foreign language fluently, maybe it's so you can take your children on a trip abroad and make their experience even more enriching. If you want to go back to school to get a degree, it's probably so you can have a new profession or re-enter the work force, doing something meaningful that helps create something for the world or helps people solve a problem.

Having a "why" keeps you focused on your goal when you feel like giving up. If your goal affects not just you but those around you (or all of humanity) you're going to push through feelings of inadequacy, fear, discomfort, and discouragement and keep going.

How to set your big goal

So now let's look at the exact process for setting your big goal. This is the fun part!

1. Get a journal. Go to a coffee shop and sit down with no distractions or interruptions. This is your time, your hour where you're not doing anything for anyone but yourself.

2. Write down every single dream you ever had as a young girl, even if you're not sure you still want it. Don't judge yourself, and don't try to write it perfectly. Just let it rip, especially the dreams that seem outlandish or crazy. If you wanted to be an astronaut, write it down.

3. Choose the three that set your heart on fire. (And if it's being an astronaut — awesome!)

4. Circle the one that is a combination of achievable for where you are in your life right now and also scary. Only you know which one that is.

5. On a separate page, write down every single action you could take to make that dream a reality. Write down the big actions and the small ones. Take the bigger action steps and break those down into teeny, tiny baby steps.

6. Order the steps from those that are easy to immediately take action on to those that would be the most challenging to act on.

7. As soon as you leave the coffee shop, take the first action. And if you can't do it right that second, write it in your day planner and check it off as soon as possible.

8. Resolve to take action on three items on the list per week — but shoot for one every single day. Be nice to yourself when life gets in the way. But stay focused.

9. Never, ever give up until the goal is achieved, no matter how long it takes.

Remember that there can be multiple phases of a big dream. If you wanted to climb Mt. Everest when you were a girl, and going from the carpool line to being Sir Edmund Hillary is out of the question (at least for now), set a goal of climbing a mountain that's closer to home.

If you dreamed of being an interpreter for the United Nations, you don't have to get your resume ready. But set a goal to speak a language you love fluently — and plan a trip to visit a country that speaks that language. (Then dust off your resume. I don't care if you just turned 40 and have three small children — if you set a goal to work for the UN, there's absolutely no reason you can't achieve it.)

Again, you want your goal to be scary enough to generate excitement and anticipation but not so out of the realm that you defeat yourself before you even get started. Once you do this long enough, you'll start to increase the size and scope of your dreams.

———————

Remember that losing weight isn't what you're after — it's the life you imagine living once you lose the weight. And that life can be yours if you just set an exciting, fulfilling goal and start working toward it.

Finding Your Voice

It took me quite a long time to develop a voice,
and now that I have it I am not going to be silent.
— Madeleine Albright

If you've come this far, you've figured out by now that this whole book is about more than losing weight — that weight isn't even the real problem.

You know that my main message is that you need to stop wasting your life trying to lose weight. You should be living your most beautiful life first, focused on achieving a bigger goal and working toward it, and naturally lose weight in the process.

But there's an even deeper message that I want to get across.

I've been saying throughout the book that the weight is only a symptom of the problem and that the real problem is how you eat.

Now what I want you to get is that spending enormous amounts of time and energy working tirelessly to lose weight and obsessing about losing it is also a symptom of a bigger problem.

And it's this: silencing your voice.

The fact that women everywhere are going through the motions of their lives without really living because the persistent thought in the back of their minds is that they need to lose weight, and the fact that they spend their days hating what they look like and devising plans to fix themselves from the outside in, is all a direct result of a collective cultural brainwashing that tells women to be quiet.

Women are taught practically from day one to silence their voices. There are varying levels of this, depending on the community you live in and the family you were raised by, but the message that women shouldn't speak with their authentic voices permeates our culture.

Maybe you were raised in a home where you were taught that you should be strong and brave and that your ambitions were to be celebrated and that you should be confident and speak up and say it loudly. If you were, you were one of the lucky ones. And if you are, you probably don't obsess about your body, if you even think about it at all.

But if you picked up this book and are still reading it, I'm going to make the leap and assume that this isn't you.

Even if you were raised in a home where you were encouraged to develop into a strong, confident woman, you were still raised in a society where women are taught that the most important thing we have to offer is our looks. And if you are inordinately focused on them — to the exclusion of becoming who you were meant to be — you are on some level silencing your inner voice.

This manifests in hundreds of ways, including working ceaselessly to look good and attempting to stay flawlessly beautiful, however old you are.

You see women silencing their voices when they put themselves down. When they say "sorry" for every little thing. When they let people (mostly men) talk over them. When they agree with people even when they secretly don't. When they move out of everyone's way. When they RSVP yes when they don't want to go.

You see them silencing themselves when they smile when they're angry. When they don't say what they're thinking for fear of offending someone else. When they defer to other people. When they never express their needs. When they don't ask for help. When they suffer in silence so they don't burden anyone. When they live a half-lived life because they're afraid their goals and dreams would inconvenience others.

I absorbed this message that I should be quiet early on. (Well-meaning, incredibly loving people can pass this message on, because it's a cultural issue and they are likely just as deeply affected by it.) My parents entertained frequently, so there were tons of people coming through our house.

I remember sitting in my living room when I was about twelve years old with my parents and five or six couples who were friends of theirs. I don't remember the exact conversation, but I remember disagreeing with what was being said. I remember trying to interject and give my opinion. No one directly shut me down, but what happened was far worse — I was completely talked over as if I hadn't said a word. It was as if I were invisible.

I also noticed that it was only the men who were talking. They were telling long, drawn-out stories, congratulating each other, and reiterating what had already been said a hundred times. Not one woman uttered a word the entire time. They all sat quietly, sipping on their drinks. I remember feeling a quiet rage that the women weren't saying anything. It was painful to watch them enduring this pointless display of male entitlement, of it being a given that the men had the floor and that they would dominate the entire conversation — if you could even call it that.

This kind of scene repeated itself constantly. On another occasion, one of my dad's friends asked my father if he wanted a beer, and when my father said yes, the man turned to me and said, "Camille, run downstairs and get your dad a beer, and while you're down there, get me one, too."

Reflexively, I shot back, "Get it yourself." And rather than being appalled that a grown man would treat his daughter like a servant, my father was horrified that I would be so "rude." (Like I said, my father was also a victim of this cultural brainwashing.)

But this push-back voice, the authentic voice inside me, didn't last long. I was taught to defer to the male voice around me — in whatever form it took — and never be disrespectful enough to challenge it. At the same time, I wondered why I had such a visceral reaction to episodes like that. I wondered what was wrong with me, certain that it was me.

So, I did what I would continue to do for years to come. I swallowed all that rage and left it nowhere to go but straight to my heart. I focused all my attention on what I was being trained to be: a good girl. And I was *really* good at it.

A good girl doesn't demand anything. She doesn't speak up, and she doesn't talk back. She doesn't fight back. She doesn't get angry, and she doesn't offend people. She doesn't challenge other people's opinions. She doesn't get what she needs, because she never asks for what she needs.

A good girl is quiet, demure, unobtrusive, and inoffensive. She agrees with whatever's being said. She makes everyone around her comfortable, even if she's not. She doesn't take up space. She defers to others and denies herself.

And above all, a good girl always, *always* looks good.

You may not have had as extreme of a takeaway as I did growing up, but I'll bet you received some of these same messages to one degree or another.

The problem with silencing yourself this way is that you're rejecting your authentic self. Your inner voice is your authentic self, expressing itself. So, when you consistently keep yourself quiet — and do it for years and years — your authentic self eventually stops making itself known.

But if you keep silencing your authentic self long enough, her voice turns into rage. And that rage ultimately gets expressed inwardly — you turn all that rage on yourself.

And what happens then? Rejecting your authentic self causes a disconnect. You can't reject your authentic self and not suffer consequences. So, if you keep suppressing your pain and anger because you've been taught that it's socially unacceptable to express it, you'll end up neutralizing it with whatever you can find — in this case, food.

But doing what we're taught to do, silencing ourselves and standing on the sidelines as nothing more than pretty accessories, eventually becomes too much, so we eat to numb the pain. And the irony is that shoving down food makes us failures at the one goal we've been conditioned to achieve at all costs: look good. So, even though we did everything we were told to do, we end up failing anyway. You have to not only be good, you have to look good while you're doing it.

This is how we keep ourselves locked in a prison of silence and rage, eating to make it go away, feeling shame because we failed, and working around the clock to cover up the evidence of our failure. We spend our lives trying to alter ourselves from the outside in, just like we were taught to. And it doesn't even look insane, because everyone around us is doing it, too.

But what if women just started speaking and living authentically? Once you start acknowledging that inner voice and letting it speak, it obliterates everything you've been taught to believe about yourself — all of the lies about how you should act and how "good" you should be.

It also obliterates the biggest lie of all: that the best you can hope for

201

in this life is to be attractive — that you are here solely for the approval of other people.

Once you start living from your authentic self, you start to care less — a lot less — about what you look like. This doesn't mean that you stop caring at all. It just means that you start caring because of how it makes you feel and not because of how other people will perceive you.

When you make this shift, you start naturally gravitating toward good habits, and the destructive habits you're trying so hard to get rid of become less appealing and eventually go away. You stop picking your body apart, hating what you see, and start loving every single thing about yourself, including the way you look.

You start seeing yourself from the inside out rather than the outside in. And the urge to binge evaporates — because there's no need to shove food down when you're no longer shoving down your voice.

When you start letting yourself speak, when you start letting who you really are emerge, you won't believe how your life will change. You probably aren't even aware of who you really are and who you're capable of becoming because you've been quiet for so long.

At age 50, I am finally dismantling the be good/look good narrative and finding my true voice. And to find it, I've had to upend many of the roles I played and the expectations other people had of me. I've had to say no to parts of my life that were socially and culturally acceptable but which caused me deep pain as a result of living inauthentically. I've learned to say what is true for me and not justify it or explain it.

And it hasn't been easy. It has been extraordinarily painful — but also totally liberating. It's like skydiving: the excruciating terror you feel at jumping out of the plane is nothing compared to the exhilaration of the freefall in the clear blue sky.

Living authentically and finally letting your real self emerge takes practice. You're not going to wake up and become a new person overnight — and you're also not going to upend your whole life, giving everyone around you the middle finger. (Or maybe you will. I fully support this.)

Actually, when you start speaking up, your relationships with other people become better because you'll feel more fulfilled when you insist on having your opinions heard, your feelings expressed, and your needs met. Most importantly, the relationship you have with yourself will become sacred, and you'll honor it and start treating yourself and your body with the utmost respect.

You'll immediately see how oppressive and soul-destroying the weight of trying to be perfect is, and you'll instantly recognize that the weight you carry on your body is in direct proportion to the level of perfection you've been striving for.

So, start letting yourself speak. Say no. Don't explain yourself. Don't justify your actions. Whatever you're feeling, calmly express it. Say what you need to say.

If you don't want to go, don't. If you don't feel like talking, don't. If you need time to yourself, take it. If you're sick of it, walk away. And if you're angry, let it out.

If you're worried what everyone will say, do it anyway. And if you think it's really going to rock the boat, then definitely do it.

Don't move out of the way. Don't say sorry unless you really mean it. Don't smile if you don't feel like it. Don't try to make everyone else feel comfortable.

Don't suck it in. Don't cover it up. Don't talk about how fat you look. Don't talk about how you look at all.

Stop feeling "less than." Stop pretending to be someone you're not. Stop living a small life. Stop wasting your life obsessing about how much you weigh.

Inhabit your body. Take up space. Speak up and insist on being heard.

Acknowledge who you really are and who you're capable of becoming.

Set a big goal and start taking action. Believe in a cherished dream and don't let anyone crush it.

Love who you were, who you are, and who you'll become.

Love your life and love yourself on every level.

Do this, and — I promise you — the weight will lose itself.

Acknowledgments

There are several people I'd like to thank who helped me, directly or indirectly, get this book published:

To Ellen Taratus, who did the final edits, thank you for improving my book and most of all for being such a good friend.

To Malina Jacobowitz, thank you for doing the beautiful cover design and for being so patient with all my changes.

To my friend Brooke Lowry, fellow book writer, thank you for being "my only friend in Charlotte" and for all your support this past year.

To my Georgia girlfriends, Katherine Buckner, Amy Chandler, Jeannie Haden, Charlotte White, Jenny Brinkley, Erin Gray, Kim Turner, and Tina Carpenter, thank you for your blog post comments, social media likes, and encouraging texts and phone calls that always keep me going.

To my new neighbor and friend Lynn Shearon, I'm so grateful I moved next door to you.

To Frannie Martin, thank you for showing me unconditional love and what true kindness looks like.

To Celeste Orr and Erin Avery, my connection to the new entrepreneurial life I'm creating, thank you both for your encouragement and your support of my new business.

To Marie Forleo and Glennon Doyle, who have no idea who I am but who inspire me every day with their work.

To my brother, Kent Smith, and my sister-in-law, Stephanie Smith, thank you for always being there for me and for making me laugh no matter what is happening.

To my parents, Myrna and Loran Smith, who have supported me in every way for the last fifty years. Thank you for being the most loving parents and grandparents ever and for modeling the kind of adventurous and engaged life I aspire to and want to give my children. I love you so much, and I could never repay you for everything you've done for me.

For Rocky Novellino, whose love has transformed me into the woman I was always meant to be. I love you with all my heart.

Most of all to Sophie and Penny, for being patient and giving up hours of "mom" time while I wrote and rewrote. I'm so grateful to be your mother and your guide in this life. This book is for you, in the hope that you will be inspired not only by its message but also by watching your mother put it out into the world, knowing that you can do anything, too. Don't let anyone ever dim your little light, always be exactly who you are, no matter what anyone else thinks, and live the life you were born to live. I love you.

For more information, inspiration,
and motivation, sign up for my blog at

camillemartinrd.com

Love To Lose
Love Your Life | Lose the Weight

Made in the USA
Columbia, SC
02 July 2020

11604495R00129